D1326020

What Would You Do?

WHAT WOULD YOU DO?

Juggling Bioethics and Ethnography

CHARLES L. BOSK

The University of Chicago Press

Chicago and London

Charles L. Bosk is professor of sociology at the University of Pennsylvania and the author of *Forgive and Remember: Managing Medical Failure* and *All God's Mistakes: Genetic Counseling in a Pediatric Hospital,* both published by the University of Chicago Press.

The University of Chicago Press, Chicago 60637
The University of Chicago Press, Ltd., London
© 2008 by The University of Chicago
All rights reserved. Published 2008
Printed in the United States of America

17 16 15 14 13 12 11 10 09 08   1 2 3 4 5

ISBN-13: 978-0-226-06676-9 (cloth)
ISBN-13: 978-0-226-06677-6 (paper)
ISBN-10: 0-226-06676-2 (cloth)
ISBN-10: 0-226-06677-0 (paper)

Library of Congress Cataloging-in-Publication Data

Bosk, Charles L.
    What would you do? : juggling bioethics and ethnography / Charles Bosk.
        p. ; cm.
    Includes bibliographical references and index.
    ISBN-13: 978-0-226-06676-9 (cloth : alk. paper)
    ISBN-10: 0-226-06676-2 (cloth : alk. paper)
    ISBN-13: 978-0-226-06677-6 (paper : alk. paper)
    ISBN-10: 0-226-06677-0 (paper : alk. paper)
    1. Bioethics. 2. Ethnology. I. Title.
    [DNLM: 1. Bioethics—Essays. 2. Anthropology, Cultural—Essays. WB 60 B743w 2008]
    QH332.B72 2008
    174'.957—dc22

                                                    2007044146

♾ The paper used in this publication meets the minimum requirements of the American National Standard for Information Sciences—Permanence of Paper for Printed Library Materials, ANSI Z39.48-1992.

For Marjorie
If this book were a movie
The credits would read
Producer and Co-Director

Contents

ACKNOWLEDGMENTS

This book has encountered multiple delays in the publication process. Each of these delays only served to increase the number of people who made its eventual appearance possible. The delays also have heightened the risk that I will omit a name, fail to provide a necessary expression of gratitude for an unexpected act of kindness and generosity, and unintentionally slight someone dear to me. If this occurs, I hope who ever is slighted forgives me quickly and does not remember the offense for too long.

There are a number of institutions, ad hoc task forces and committees, and foundations that provided the occasion for writing and an audience for critiquing the first draft of the essays that appear here.

The Social Science and Humanities Research Council of Canada, the now-defunct Westminster Institute of Canada, and the University of Western Ontario provided the funds and Barry Hoffmaster provided the organizational genius for a series of meetings over two years for a project titled "Humanizing Bioethics." The first drafts of "A Sociologist's Apology, a Bioethicist's Lament: The Surgeon and the Sociologist Revisited," "Irony, Ethnography, and Informed Consent," and "A Monument of Silence: On Not Giving Up Dr. Arthur's Ghost" were all written over the period this group was meeting regularly.

Members of this group included Renee Anspach, Diane Beeson, Michael Burgess, Peter Conrad, Sydney Halpern, Barry Hoffmaster, Bruce Jennings, Sharon Kauffman, Barbara Koenig, Margaret Lock, Kate McBurney, Patty Marshall, and Alison Wylie. The chance to discuss the intersection of social science multiple times over a period of a couple of years with these colleagues was a rare and wonderful experience. It continues to inform my work in ways large and small.

The Greenwall Foundation supported a working group of social scientists, bioethicists, and physicians at the University of Pennsylvania. This allowed me my first opportunity to revise each of those essays. Colleagues who deserve special thanks for their participation as part of this group include Robbie Aronowitz, Art Caplan, Donald Light, Jon Merz, Pamela Sankar, Miriam Solomon, and Peter Ubel. I am especially grateful to Jacqueline Hart and Sita Reddy, who organized these meetings and provided critical readings of my revised efforts.

The Greenwall Foundation also supported the Task Force on Guidelines and Standards for Ethics Consultation of the American Society for Bioethics and Humanities. The essay "The Licensing and Certification of Ethics Consultants: What Part of "No!" Was So Hard to Understand?" was written as a consequence of my having had the opportunity to discuss the issues surrounding the organization of ethics over a period of a couple of years with a thoughtful group of colleagues drawn from multiple disciplines who provided consultation services in regionally dispersed and institutionally diverse health care organizations ranging from rural nursing homes to urban academic medical centers. I am grateful to Robert Arnold and Stewart Youngner for inviting me to join the group and to Mark Aulisio for organizing our meetings in such a thoughtful way. All of the members of the Task Force helped me recognize how plural the practice of bioethics is at the bedside. The Greenwall Foundation also provided support for a working group on medical error and a conference at the School of Public Health at the University of California, Berkeley. My participation with the group and at the conference provided the impetus for "Margin of Error: The Sociology of Ethics Consultation."

A conference at the University of Michigan underwritten by the American Sociological Association under its Future of the Discipline program provided the opportunity to think yet again about the multiplicity of ways that rise of visible ethical concerns in the provision of clinical care and in issues of science and health care policy. Robert Zussman organized the conference and Carl Schneider and Renee Anspach hosted it. An opportunity to refine my thinking on paper was presented by Art Kleinman and the Department of Social Medicine at Harvard during the first Rivers Conference on Medical Ethics.

The Introduction to this volume, "What Would You Do? Juggling Bioethics and Ethnography," the conclusion, "Professional Expertise and Moral Cowardice: Counterfeit Courage and the Noncombatant," as well as "Bureaucracies of Mass Deception: Institutional Review Boards and the Ethics of Ethnographic Research" (coauthored with Raymond G. De Vries) are products of an academic leave for 2003–4 during which I was in residence at the School of Social Science at the Institute for Advanced Study, Princeton, New Jersey. I am grateful to seminar participants for much more than their comments when I presented a draft of "Professional Expertise and Moral Cowardice" in the seminar on bioethics. The opportunity to spend a year in the company of Philippe Bourgois, Tod Chambers, Louis Charland, Joe Davis, Ray De Vries, Carl Eliot, Trudo Leemans, Adriana Petryna, Leigh Turner, Elizabeth Wilson, and Noam Zohar was a wondrous gift. I would like to thank the School of Arts and Sciences at the University of Pennsylvania for allowing me to place my leave account temporarily in arrears so that I was able to receive this gift. Institute faculty—the late Cliff Geertz, Eric Maskin, Joan Scott, and Michael Walzer—provided encouragement through a balance of skepticism and support. Harold Shapiro's perspective in the seminar as the former chair of the president's National Bioethics Advisory Commission constantly reminded of just how plural a noun bioethics is.

At one time or another I received comments on the drafts of various of the papers collected here from a long list of colleagues over such a long period of time that listing them risks not giving a colleague credit where credit is due. Friends and colleagues who provided useful suggestions and who have not previously been named include Howie Becker, Harold Bershady, Alan Brandt, Richard Cook, Mary-Jo DelVecchio Good, Robert Dingwall, Norm Fost, the late Eliot Freidson, Carol Heimer, Joel Howell, Al Jonsen, Rosemary Stevens, David Rothman, Charles Rosenberg, Sue Rubin, Susan Watkins, Eviatar Zerubavel, and Laurie Zoloth. Barbara Katz Rothman scribbled the book's interrogatory title on a napkin during lunch at the Institute.

I lean on certain colleagues for feedback more than others. Renee Fox has for a very long time been a source of valuable feedback, warning me away from overly glib formulations with just the right gentle question or arch of the eyebrow. Joel Frader and Carla Keirns have been responsible in very large part for my continuing medical education. To them has fallen an onerous task that they handled with great patience and humor. Elizabeth Armstrong and Joanna Kempner have proved as relentless as critics of my prose as I have been of theirs. Mark Jacobs has been a source of sound practical and editorial advice from the beginning of graduate school to the present. Whenever I am not certain about what I am doing or whether whatever I am writing is worth the trouble, I turn to Mark, whose replies for more than thirty years have been excessive in their speed and thoughtfulness. Margaret Ensminger and Jim Lynch have always responded whenever I have asked for help.

At the University of Chicago Press, Doug Mitchell has been a constant source of encouragement, Tim McGovern shepherded this book through the production process, and Rebecca Sullivan's careful editing improved the text. At the University of Pennsylvania, Carolanne Saunders helped with the assembly of the final manuscript. Jane Ballerini spent part of a summer internship assembling and checking references.

An academic, I live a large portion of my life inside my head, and I am very thankful to a large network of family and friends who welcome me when I wander into the world. My daughters, Emily and Abigail, have learned to tolerate those moments when I am bodily present but somewhere else. My wife, Marjorie, cannot be adequately thanked in a sentence. She is, and has always been, a model of and a model for personal and intellectual honesty. Over the years she has taught me the importance of always probing one level deeper.

What Would You Do?

JUGGLING BIOETHICS AND ETHNOGRAPHY

I like to think of myself as a responsible member of the academic community. Yet on rereading essays that I have written, I noticed that they were so carelessly assembled that I had committed the offense of academic littering. All of this littering indicated that I was in the grip of that strange academic syndrome, *dysdouglassia*—I had left a lot of matter out of place. With the most innocent of intentions, I had created a mess.

This is a first, fumbling attempt of a sociological fox to behave more like a hedgehog, to borrow Isaiah Berlin's characterization of intellectual styles. The gathering, repackaging, and reframing of previously published essays (and more than a few unpublished ones) is my humble effort to contribute to a more sustainable commons in the environment shared by bioethicists, ethnographers, health care providers, health services researchers, and all those concerned with policy at a micro or macro level. A criterion for judging whether the personal recycling policy adopted here is worth the expenditure of the nonsustainable energy that has been invested in producing it is this: that these essays are "good to think with," that is, that they add resources to the public discourse of ethical dilemmas inherent in clinical medicine or the attempt to do research either within or on the domain of medical research.

The essays collected here juggle two themes: (1) the emergent social organization of the everyday ethical dilemmas of clinical care and medical research as a distinct domain, organized by experts in bioethics—I look at an emergent cadre of workers with a sociological eye and (2) the everyday ethical problems I experience as an observer, and sometimes participant, doing ethnography, living among bioethicists, health care providers, health services researchers, and policy makers—I look at the everyday, taken-for-granted practices of the ethnographic researcher and try to view those through the lens of ethics. What holds these essays together is the attempt to take ethics seriously as a form of organized behavior within health care or as social process—a set of recurrent problems that I experience either when I am "in the field" gathering data or "at the table" being asked to proffer an expert opinion. What is being juggled is my viewpoint—there is something to be gained from looking at the sleight of hand involved in this juggling—what are the differences found when I am attempting to understand the bio-ethicist as "other" and the ethnographer as "other"? Because we are all aware of how limited in practice our abilities are to stand beside ourselves and view our behavior as others do, the outlandish promises of theories that discuss "looking-glass selves" notwithstanding, I would forgive any gentle readers a very intense skepticism about whether the juggling that these essays promise is possible if they would but willingly suspend their disbelief long enough to allow me to explain how I came to do this juggling. To do this, I need to explain the title and the organization of this volume twice: not as tragedy and farce but as theory and narrative.

What Would You Do?

The first part of the title, *What Would You Do?* is a question that I encounter frequently in the clinical domains where I conduct my research. I hear the question first as an expression of anguish, the *angst* of appearing to have few acceptable options. I hear the question second as a request for guidance in decision making, a plea for someone to exercise the *agency* necessary to make choices within the narrow range of acceptable options. When one is a legitimate agent, then one is entitled to take *action*. What does it mean to experience angst? How in the face of angst does one exercise agency? What does it mean to take responsibility for action? I think and write about those questions on the basis of my experience as an ethnographer in academic hospitals in the last quarter of the twentieth century and the opening years of the twenty-first century. As an empirical social scientist, I define angst and agency operationally as they are acted out in social life.

The operational definitions that I use to research these questions overlap imperfectly with both those of social actors who must in the moment define situations as if they were real (because, well, in the moment they are) and live with the consequences of those decisions and those of bioethicists who attempt to provide clarity on who is and who is not a legitimate agent, who is or is not entitled to take action, and what action legitimate agents are permitted to take or prohibited from taking. I define angst as a recurrent moment in social life when moral uncertainty, interpersonal conflict, or collective anxieties derail smooth social interaction. I define agency as the fix that allows action to move, however tentatively or assertively, over uncertain tracks through uncharted terrain. I define action as a sequence of bundled behaviors that results in an outcome that is fodder for measurement, assessment, comparison, and improvement.

As an ethnographer, I look for the experience of angst as occurring in a primal social moment: when a troubled decision-maker turns to another and asks, "What would you do in my situation?" I view this question as an indicator of decision making halted, hear it as an index of organizational troubles, and feel it as a set of crisscrossing tensions, a web of misunderstood and often conflicting agendas, a signal of a network of potential problems—clinical, administrative, legal, and political. As an ethnographer I have both watched and witnessed this question asked of others many times. I have heard patients facing risky surgery and even-riskier nonsurgical options ask it of their surgeons. I have heard parents of pediatric intensive care patients ask it of treatment team members—nurses, social workers, interns and residents, fellows, and attending physicians—as well as of each other. I have heard couples facing excruciatingly complex and terrifying reproductive choices ask it of genetic counselors. I have heard physicians ask it of colleagues whose opinion they sought before they either cautiously extended a toe or plunged headlong into troubled waters. I have heard nurses ask it of other nurses when confronted with questionable physician behavior. I have heard residents ask it of other residents when contemplating challenging the authority of attending physicians. I think of these situations as moments of *clinical angst.*

Clinical angst is an everyday experience for many workers in academic medical centers faced with answering those questions that Weber discussed in "Science as a Vocation." These are questions where the approach of a "natural scientist" will not yield a solution to the problem of "whether life is worthwhile living and when." As Weber points out, while natural science provides answers for how "to master life technically, it leaves quite aside or assumes for its purposes, whether we should wish and do wish to master life technically and whether it makes ultimate sense to do so" (Weber in Gerth and Mills 1946, 144).

As an ethnographer, I have not just watched others answer the question "What would you do if you were in my situation?"—I have often been asked for an answer to this question myself. It is a question that invariably plunges me into an existential and moral panic. My responses to the question model nothing so much as hesitation, doubt, and uncertainty. I am at sea. I have no particular expertise upon which I feel qualified to give normative advice in clinical situations. I identify these moments as *ethnographic angst*. I am a researcher. What I think I would do is irrelevant. I have been trained not to give advice. To do so is to violate the rules of my role. All of these considerations do not mean that I always forego giving advice. There are moments when uncertain and wavering cognitive and normative barriers are breached. Violations are noticed or ignored. The everyday work life of the group goes on. I work with these people (or, at the least, hope they will tolerate my living among them for a time so I can understand them later); I can't be both a part of ongoing group life and as silent as a stone. My responses satisfy or disappoint. They exert an unseen influence on what the group does, what it allows me to see, when it chooses to ask my advice again and for what.

The perils, pains, and pressures of clinical angst are now ritual routines of organized behavior: bureaucratized and socially organized as clinical definitions, procedures, guidelines, rules, and formal regulations. A few are even identified and codified in official documents as "best practices." The set of socially visible practices that we identify as clinical bioethics are designed to anaesthetize patients and their families and health care workers to the dreadful ethical decisions required as part of everyday practice in the academic medical center pioneering new frontiers in clinical care. The deadening of feeling is, perhaps, a requirement for certain sorts of decisions and actions: the decision to withdraw support from a patient so that the harvesting of organs can begin at the narrow portal betwixt life and death is a particularly vivid example.

One task for the ethnographer of hospital life is to watch and witness the transformation of the perils, pains, and pressures of terrifying choices into bureaucratic routines, describe this transformation as richly as possible from the point of view of as many stakeholders as can be held in one's head at one time, record them in field notes, and present them to colleagues as accounts of social process. No matter how extraordinary are the decision making and actions of those providing medical care, everyday role responsibilities dampen clinical angst for those involved; everyday responsibilities of ethnographers require its amplification, the better to recapture the awesome nature of exactly what choices have been so routinely bureaucratized. One of the offices of ethnography is to re-enchant disenchanted modernity—all the better to recapture the quotidian horrors that we take for granted as normal or natural.

In the crucible of everyday decision making, clinical angst is managed through an organizational structure of role-defined responsibilities. There is the need to get on with things. The question "What should we do now in this situation?" demands an answer. Other work and problems always exert a pressure to do something, to make a decision, to act. However, for the ethnographer, nothing save the need to establish rapport, build trust, and participate in the ongoing life of the group justifies answering this question. These are, of course, powerful justifications: without establishing rapport, building trust and participating in the ongoing life of the group, ethnographic study is not possible.

As a field-worker, I seek medical settings where "What would you do in my situation?" is most likely to be asked. To wax philosophical, clinical angst is nothing less than my ethnographic reason for being, or, more properly, my reason for choosing to be here or there, at this or that field site, at this or that time, with these or those people. Primarily, I want to understand, describe, and explain how these professionals ask and answer this question of each other. I have long been interested in how, in the occupational community of physicians, collective professional responsibility is understood and enacted in the instance and in the breach. I see as well how lay participants ask these questions and how they respond to professional answers to them. For the purposes of observation, "What would you do if you were in my situation?" is an orienting question; it involves a bounded whole of others, whose trained competencies and role responsibilities are different from my own. I provide situated explanations of how health care workers define and manage questions that the work group categorizes as "ethical" or as "our responsibility." These explanations are the solution to a sociological puzzle, a game of rules and roles, interpreted, followed, and evaded. I am not a player of this game. I record the moves of others, catalogue the outcomes, analyze the strategies, imagine how outcomes might have been otherwise had different moves and strategies been adopted, and wonder what would have happened if other games with other rules had been played.

If clinical angst orients actors with defined role responsibilities in the situation—doctor, nurse, ethicist, parent—and if those role responsibilities then guide action, then *ethnographic angst* has the opposite effect on field-workers: it disorients. Being asked directly, "Well, what would you do?" dissolves all frames for analyzing interaction that leave the ethnographer out of the picture, outside the frame of the action described. Being called upon to venture an opinion raises for me a set of existential questions. How I answer the question answers as well: Why am I here in this setting and what do I think I am doing?

When I am in the field, working, gathering data, the question "What would you do in this situation?" disrupts the main pose that I am attempting to sustain as an ethnographer. That main pose is a fantastic *fictio* that I am unseen, observing but unobserved, that my presence changes things in no way that is significant enough to notice. Taking the question "What would you do?" seriously requires that I consider the possibility that my being there makes a difference to the way action unfolds. If this is so, the central conceit of participant observation as I try to do it collapses: namely, the conceit that results are valid because observer effects are minimal.

I have stated that I am at sea largely because I do not know how to provide a well-formed professional answer to the question "What would you do if you were in my situation?" It is not that I am empty of strong opinions. However, when I ask to be allowed to observe settings, one of my opening promises to the group is that I will disturb things as little as possible. Answering the question "What would you do?" the moment it is put always feels like a breaking of that promise. Following Weber, there are questions to which even if we were "to master life technically" neither the natural nor social sciences provide an answer. The ethnographic social scientist, who provides an answer to these questions as they unfold in clinical settings, has created the awkward stylistic requirement that this answer now needs to be described as objectively, as impersonally, as all the others. The ethnographer's answer enters into the social process ; it is one among many voices that shaped how angst was resolved, agency legitimated, and action taken. However skilled ethnographers may be at viewing themselves as others would, the ethnographer has no reason to expect that readers will take claims either of neutrality or even virtuous advocacy that saved the day seriously. All ethnographers know that the accounts of the partisans in action are accepted with great skepticism. Clinical angst refers then to those situations in which hospital workers ask each other what is to be done; ethnographic angst refers to situations in which as a technical expert on social behavior doing empirical research, I am asked to resolve a normative question. It refers to those moments immediately before providing the requested help or, more commonly, refraining from doing so.

Agency refers to how surgeons, genetic counselors, and clinical bioethicists act when asked "What would you do if you were in my situation?"

For surgeons in the mid-1970s, there were decisions that "only an attending can make." Among these were deciding whether to intervene, and, if so, what kind of intervention to make. For genetic counselors in the early years of the 1980s, the question, whether asked by colleagues or lay clients, elicited a string of questions in return. Each question sought with ever-sharper clarity a definition of what "your situation is exactly." For clinical bioethicists in the late 1990s, the question was a clear signal that clinical consultations needed to take place, policies needed to be promulgated, principles needed following, processes needed facilitation, stakeholders needed education, and resolutions needed ratification.

Action is both the bundled behaviors and the outcome of those behaviors that are initiated by a legitimate agent. As our interest in assessing outcomes and in taking active measures to improve them grows, and grow it will, if only because of the need to manage responsibly and allocate efficiently scarce and expensive health care resources, attention is likely to turn even more intensively than it already has to questions of which agents are likely to make the best decisions in what kind of situations.

Juggling Bioethics and Ethnography

The first part of the title describes a sequence of behavior. The second part describes an activity—juggling—for formulating, refining, deepening, and probing the everyday ethical dilemmas that emerge from a sustained engagement with bioethics as a sociologist who does ethnographic research. I have so far argued that ethnographers are condemned to experience intense angst in clinical situations because they must refrain from exercising clinical agency. This position will receive fuller elaboration in the chapters that follow. Here I want to provide a spare outline of the reasons behind it, indicate that I am aware of the multiple alternatives to this view of defining role responsibilities, and describe how this position evolved as I did firsthand observational research in a variety of medical settings.

I have stated that I think ethnographers in medical settings should not volunteer an answer to the question "What would you do in this situation?"—that, in general, indirect evasion is to be preferred to decisive forthrightness. For the sake of clarity, I should be slightly more specific. While in the field, as a study is going forward, we should refrain from answering the question "What would you do?" whenever possible. Once we are freed from the exigencies of gathering data, different rules apply. After all, the question itself is of intense interest to us as field-workers. My writing up of my field experiences is often an extended meditation on the question "What would you do?" The meditation first describes how others, especially those others who were in the seat of judgment, answered the question for themselves, a meditation on what they did and their rationales for action. As a meditation on the answers and responses that those in that seat of judgment provided in situations of risky choice under time pressures and irreducible uncertainty, my writing seeks to sort out the complexities embedded in action, point out the costs and benefits of various responses, and, at the end of the day, make some judgments about which costs are worth incurring and which are not, as well as which benefits are worth the associated costs and which ought to be foregone. Sociological interpretations of action are never free from this sort of normative freight; nor ought they be. However, the normative chip I wear on my shoulder while doing fieldwork is one that I try to display as unobtrusively as possible.

The reasons that I adopt this pose are many. Answering the question "What would you do?" either too hastily or too decisively cuts off the flow of talk and feeling of actors in the setting. This flow of talk and expression of feeling is precisely what ethnographers seek to capture so that there might be some data to analyze later. As a practical matter, ethnographers ought to do as little as possible to cut off the social action that they are most interested in describing. Second, ethnographers generally have little pragmatic training or theoretic knowledge to guide intervention in situations of conflict. I do not necessarily believe that such training provides for better or worse outcomes. What it does allow is a plausible claim of technical expertise sufficient to justify intervention. The putative expert has a rationale for being here and having been asked to do this or that. The fact that such expertise provides uncertain legitimation, that those who use their expertise to act may act mistakenly or that their expertise is open to challenge, is a major theme of the essays in Part One of this volume. Nonetheless, however uncertain or illegitimate the expertise that justifies intervention of others, it has been articulated in a way that fits some role-bound definition of rights, duties, and responsibilities. This is simply not so for ethnographers of uncertain medical action in situations of risky choice.

Finally, to act too decisively or too frequently is to engage in some action other than doing ethnography. That action may be praiseworthy, may contribute much to the common good, and may have more value than ethnographic description. This is not the issue. However, being a too-visible actor with a too-established point of view makes claims of impartial description, claims that are difficult enough to sustain as it is, impossible to take seriously. To advocate too vigorously for any solution to the question "What would you do in this situation?" may be to engage in morally necessary, virtuous action on behalf of helpless others who need aid. At the same time, a too forcefully argued position eliminates the possibility of a serious ethnography of the recurrent problems of everyday life that this group of actors faces.

My insistence here that the ethnographer not be an active participant in whatever scenes he or she describes in order to sustain the possibility of a more rigorously objective description may strike the reader abreast of current trends in ethnographic writing as somewhat odd. First, the faith of social scientists in a rigorously objective qualitative analysis is somewhat tattered, and that tattering is not without considerable justification. As a consequence, ethnographic work has become more self-reflexive in recent years. Instead of objectivity as a goal, we have transparency. If the researcher can tell us enough about his or her biases, preconceptions, preoccupations, enough about how his or her prior experiences led to the selection of this problem in this setting at this time, and enough about his or her feelings and reactions as observations were being made, then we readers can judge for ourselves how much of an ethnographic account we should trust and how much we should view skeptically. Advocates of auto-ethnography, who make plausible claims that certain types of experience can only be captured by intense self-observation, description, explanation, and analysis, are but one indicator of how little objectivity as a goal of inquiry is prized.

But I need not look to contemporary trends within ethnographic writing to find my insistence on meeting with silence the question "What would you do in this situation?" hard to justify. At the time that I first started doing fieldwork in the early years of the 1970s, a number of alternatives to the model of field-worker as objective reporter were available. An insistence on silence was an extreme response. After all, advocacy and participation action research celebrated the role of the researcher as a change agent, a positive force for social good. I was drawn to these models when I first entered the field, so I find the position that I develop through these essays personally puzzling. Aware that objectivity is an unattainable aspiration, aware that some have rejected it for models of research committed to making the world better, I found myself increasingly committed to maintaining an icy distance in the situation all the better to pursue a putatively objective description that supports a normatively freighted interpretation later, once I remove myself from the field. How did this happen?

Here is where my biography as a researcher intersects with developments in the larger society. Here is where the distinction between clinical and ethnographic angst, agency, and action has to be explained as narrative. My insistence that ethnographers in medical settings are required not to answer the question, "What would you do in this situation?" is not a conviction that, over thirty years ago, I carried with me into the field along with pen and notebook when I began to study the culture of medicine, when I looked at how physicians recognize, ignore, categorize, and respond to failure and error. Rather, it is a conviction that has developed over time; it is a conviction that has deepened as the world that I studied changed and as the expectations for what work like mine will contribute have changed as well. I realize that there is much dogmatism, some of it self-defeating, involved in taking the position that within the world of clinical ethics the ethnographic social scientist is present to experience angst and never to exercise agency or take action.

I am aware of this dogmatism because I can state this personal preference as an ethnographic first rule or principle: *The more certain the ethnographer is that exercising agency in this situation, at this moment, in this way, will relieve the angst of all parties in the situation, the more stringent is the prohibition on the ethnographer that forbids the exercise of agency.* As a first principle, "Do Nothing" runs a risk. To borrow David Rothman's phrase, with so many "strangers" at the bedside, why have another who claims to do nothing more than witness events? When "help" is needed, what of worth does a mute witness provide? I did not start with this rule—if anything, I began life as a field-worker with the reverse rule in mind. I need to sketch here how a person interested in improving social process, eager to create more social justice in the world, fashioned such a passive stance as a set of operating rules for navigating in a very complex social space. In addition, I need to explain why, when conflict arises in clinical settings, witnesses who do nothing but provide reports after the fact, are a necessary, if somewhat irritating, presence.

During the fieldwork for my book *Forgive and Remember,* I was very rarely asked what I would do in any specific situation. Ethics, as we think of it now, was not much of a concern on the Able and Baker services of Pacific Hospital. There was no great anguish around the adequacy of informed consent or the exercise of patient autonomy. Surgeons believed that the terminally ill should "die with dignity" when their time came but they also believed that it was perfectly appropriate for the surgeon to define "their time" and "dignity." There was no organized challenge to the authority of attending surgeons. Almost all conflict was subterranean. Occasionally, an attending surgeon might ask a resident or student what they would do if the patient before them were a family member. But these were not real questions, inviting real discussions. They were "set-ups" so that attending physicians might deliver little homilies on their "philosophy" of care. All but the most socially inept residents and students understood that these recitations of attending philosophy were to be heard as received wisdom and not as invitations for debate.

When attending physicians were not around, residents and students might debate amongst themselves the different philosophies of care that their teachers clung to so tenaciously. But such debates were really less about the ethics of care than the indignities of prolonged subordination. A couple of times when residents got caught up in arguments among themselves about what to do, they would ask me to judge which of them was right. On these rare occasions when I was asked what I would do, I was uncomfortable. I worried that an incorrect response might alienate someone whom I needed to gather good data from later. I tried to avoid direct answers by deflecting questions. But I do not recall any attending surgeon asking me, or anybody else, what we would do in any ethically troubled situation prospectively. In general, the more controversial the ethics of a case, the less likely it was to be a topic for public discussion.

Those cases that were perceived as ethically tangled were all the more likely on that account to be handled privately; then decisions on those cases were announced as the sort of decision that only an attending could make. Ethics were personal, ethical questions demarcated a zone where personal and professional responsibility merged and conflicted. After decision making, whatever discussion took place served only to make clear the grounds for decision making so that others might develop their own philosophy of care upon the exemplary grounds just displayed. Such discussions were not viewed as an appropriate time to explore whatever roads were not taken. Most charitably, surgeons viewed ethical discussions as a luxury that time only rarely permitted, a topic for internists who did not possess the action ethic of surgeons. Less charitably, ethical discussions were viewed as pointless diversions that served the interests of neither patient nor surgeon, as one more aggravation in a day that already contained more than enough vexations.

A scant five years passed between the conclusion of the fieldwork for *Forgive and Remember* and the initiation of fieldwork on genetic counseling for *All God's Mistakes*. I left one shop-floor environment in which clinical ethics was not a contested domain and entered one in which it was. A part of this, no doubt, was connected to the novel problems that prenatal diagnosis posed; a part, to a general trend in society to transfer decision-making authority from physicians to patients or their nearest proxies; and a part, to the emergence of bioethics as a substantive domain. The individual clinical autonomy and responsibility that so marked the behavior of surgeons was not a prominent feature of the world of genetic counselors. This was by choice. Counselors claimed that they prized client autonomy and adopted what they described as a value neutral, nondirective treatment style to achieve it. The fact that the world of the genetic counselor was different from the world of surgery was marked for me by nothing so much as the fact that genetic counselors *invited* me to study them so that they *might receive advice* on how to handle the special questions raised by their new capacities. The genetic counselors were sincerely interested in what I would do, and often not shy about asking.

At the same time that I was studying genetic counselors, I was also involved with a pediatrician, Joel Frader, and a linguist, Ellen Prince, in studies of decision making in a pediatric intensive care unit. Doctors, nurses, and parents of patients in the unit often faced the always-unsettling problem of whether or not to continue treatment. At the time there was much clinical uncertainty about whether brain death had occurred: a protocol for establishing brain death was said to exist but there was much debate about when to invoke it and what its provisions were whenever it was invoked. When issues of continuing treatment were raised in rounds, they were floated on a raft of other concerns: who should tell the parents, when did social services need to be involved, when did legal, what should be done if the parents were not ready to hear the news of brain death?

At this time, in both genetic counseling and pediatric intensive care, three interrelated developments were emerging simultaneously, although I was only dimly aware of each at the time. The interaction of each of these developments and my struggle to make sense of them both explains my increasing reluctance to respond directly to the question "What would you do if you were in my situation?" and also shapes this volume. The first and most significant development was the emergence of the ethical problem in clinical situations as a unique problem that required new procedures and new actors for its solution. The claim was often made at the time that these "ethical" dilemmas were created by new medical technologies. This view seems to ignore the fact that "ethical problems" were not a new feature of the social landscape of health care work. For example, there had long been debates about what to tell the terminally ill, when to withdraw them from treatment, and how aggressively to attempt to salvage the severely damaged. Technology, no doubt, heightened both the presence of dilemmas and awareness of them. But the rise of new technologies is not by itself a sufficient explanation for the new status of ethical problems on the shop floor of the hospital.

To these new technologies a second factor needs to be added: the erosion of trust in professional authority. Without this, new technologies are simply one more arrow in the quiver of professional authority. Without the erosion of trust, the patient is secure in the expectation that all the arrows in the physician's quiver will be aimed at the bull's eye of the patient's self-interest. For a variety of reasons, the public confidence that the physician's action would harmonize with the patient's self-interest, the public sense that they viewed a common target and shared a system for scoring how near or distant arrows landed from the center of that target dissipated in the last third of the twentieth century. I will not belabor the multiple reasons for the erosion of professional authority here since it is a major topic of Part One of this volume. All that needs to be said now is the erosion of professional authority had multiple effects: (1) it created uncertainty about where the professional decision-making authority of physicians ended and the personal decision-making authority of patients began, (2) it made clear the absence of adequate organizational solutions in those cases in which disputes arose, (3) it allowed what were formerly personal troubles of doctors and patients to enter the social arena as public issues, to name but three. How the combination of uncertain grounds upon which to base decision making, ambiguity surrounding who was empowered to make decisions, inadequate organizational processes for negotiating resolution to these ambiguities and uncertainties, and public scrutiny combined to create the professional role of bioethicist and new bureaucratic structures for managing conflict are also major themes of the essays of Part One.

A third change occurred in the organization of care that reinforced the sense of crisis in the ethics of care at the precise moment that the public trust in professional authority began to dissipate: namely, the attempt to control medical costs through a variety of strategies for managing care. The most readily observable of these strategies for controlling costs through managing care was a shift from individual insurance through employers on a fee-for-service basis to enrollment of individuals in prepaid panels of patients. The typical prepaid patient group had global budgets for patient panels. For individual patients, membership in a prepaid group made clear an inherent conflict of interest between the patient's interest in receiving care and the physician's interest in maximizing income. Individualized fee-for-service plans obscured this conflict since those patterns of over-treatment that maximize physician income also make it possible to sustain the fiction that nothing is of more value than the patient's return to health. In patient plans with global budgets, medical profit is maximized when treatment is withheld. This fact itself raises awareness of the divergence of physician and patient self-interest; it intensifies the sense that something is amiss when physicians do not accede to this or that patient's demand for a referral, a drug, or a procedure. Further, prepaid plans erode physician authority since case managers authorize many treatment plans far from the bedside.

So it was in this environment of perceived ethical crisis, erosion of patient trust in professional authority, and more explicit conflict between the self-interest of patients and the economic interests of physicians and third-party payers that I conducted the fieldwork with genetic counselors and health care workers in pediatric intensive care units. It was in this context that the question "What would you do if you were in my situation?" came up so frequently. At first, I was surprised by the frequency of the question, then I was flattered that anyone thought that my opinion might matter, and then I was angered by the frequency of the question since the various efforts to incorporate me into the group as a participant made it harder for me to do my fieldwork, made it harder for others to ignore my presence. In addition, I was both disappointed and frustrated by my inability to translate my knowledge of medical culture into pithy recommendations. I was generally a waffler. All problems had for me an "on the one hand but on the other" quality. Finally, I was frustrated by the fact that, when I could turn my insights into recommendations, when I could get off whatever fence on which I was sitting, I could find no way to do so and preserve my role as a researcher. I had neither the inclination nor the temperament to conduct participant-action research in medical settings.

At the same time, I was flabbergasted that there was emerging an inter-disciplinary group of experts—philosophers, physicians, attorneys, fellow social scientists, social workers, and theologians—who seemed to possess, publicly at least, a surer problem-solving sense than I did. I was both surprised and amazed that this new group of experts seemed as welcome in clinical settings as they did. As a sociologist, I found the emergence of this new occupational segment within health care to be both fascinating and challenging. The fascination was easy enough to understand in a medical sociologist who came to that subdiscipline through the study of work and occupations. Who were these people? From where did their sense of mission and core task come? What beliefs united them? Who was their constituency? What authority legitimated their recommendations? The challenge came from other sources—anxiety that bioethics would make the ethnographic questions that I was most interested in exploring harder to research at the same time that it created confusion over the boundary between sociology and medical ethics. There was another challenge that I did not anticipate: how to preserve an identity as a sociologist in an intellectual space that more and more defined me as either a bioethicist or an ethicist when I make no claims to be either. How were questions of culture and social structure to be kept alive in a setting that wanted to reduce all conflicts in care, whatever their structural features, to questions of "ethics" or "values"?

The essays in this volume are a response over time to my juggling the concerns of bioethics and the sensibilities of an ethnographer to take part in the world of bioethics without becoming a bioethicist. The essays are also a response to being asked so frequently, "What would you do in this situation?" They are preliminary stabs at attempting to understand more precisely what this situation is, why it is understood this way rather than that; to explore the implications of the new sets of roles and procedures that we now employ to manage those conflicts that we call "ethical"; and finally, to ask what problems are created for the ethnographer if we take questions of research ethics seriously—what does a genuine commitment to "informed consent," confidentiality, and anonymity look like? Should we judge our own work by the same standards that we impose on clinical research?

This volume is divided into three parts. Part One, "The Ethnography of Ethics" is not, strictly speaking, an ethnographic analysis. I did not conduct systematic fieldwork on how the role of bioethicist is enacted in the modern tertiary-care hospital. Rather, the essays in Part One are what survey researchers refer to as a secondary analysis. They evolved as the result of my sustained involvement within the community of bioethics and bioethicists. In that community, I have had a number of roles: faculty member in a graduate program, member of a national taskforce to examine the education and credentialing of clinical bioethicists, speaker at various conferences, author of book chapters and articles, as well as member of multiple professional societies.

Most sociologists, even most medical sociologists, are only marginally interested in the emergence of bioethics as a domain of organized activity. This domain is somewhat hard to conceptualize cleanly because it is so multiplex; I have borrowed a phrase that I first heard from Charles Rosenberg and tend to refer to the domain as that "collection of socially visible activities that we call bioethics." The collection itself is somewhat disparate. There are public-policy activities exemplified by the activities of various national and presidential commissions. There are entrepreneurial activities such as consultancies on various external advisory boards for pharmaceutical and biotech companies. There are roles within various academic institutions such as service on institutional review boards or institutional ethics committees. There is teaching and research within newly formed departments of bioethics, more often than not interdisciplinary units located within medical schools. In short, bioethics is a complex, changing interdisciplinary space that serves many masters. Increasingly, with the debates about stem cell research and the recent resurgence of concern with "right-to-die" cases such as Terri Schiavo's and the linkage of such cases with the right-to-life movement, bioethics has also become a highly politicized domain, a new battlefield in the cultural wars. The essays in Part One attempt to capture some of these dimensions of the world of bioethics. They capture as well, I hope, the tension of trying to investigate this domain of social life while trying to maintain a skeptical distance from it.

The first essay, "Professional Ethicist Available: Logical, Secular, Friendly," explores the tensions between social science analysis and bioethics. In it, I confront an initial mistaken judgment of mine. When I first encountered bioethics in 1974, the entire enterprise struck me as quixotic and surely doomed to failure. I could not have been more wrong. The essay seeks to understand why the influence of social science waned in the academic medical center as the influence of bioethics waxed. The second essay, "The Licensing and Certification of Ethics Consultants: What Part of "No!" was So Hard to Understand?" explores the dangers of thinking of "ethics expert" as a professional role like any other. The essay grows out of my participation in a national task force on the education and credentialing of clinical bioethicists. The theme that it takes up is one familiar to students of Weber, Parsons, and Freidson: how does one reconcile the claims of expert authority with the claims of autonomy, either collective or individual, in a democratic political system?

The next essay, coauthored with Joel Frader, "Institutional Ethics Committees: Sociological Oxymoron, Empirical Black Box," asks whether our enthusiasm for institutional ethics committees is misplaced. What organizational problems and paradoxes are created when we internalize the management of clinical ethics within an institution? What are institutional ethics committees created to do? How would we measure whether they are accomplishing the task? How do we separate the advocacy for such committees from research on their efficacy? The fourth essay in Part One, "Margin of Error: The Sociology of Ethics Consultation," asks whether a clinical ethicist can make a mistake. This chapter explores what it means to make a mistake within a community of practitioners. It asks whether structures of and for accountability exist within the institutional settings in which clinical consultation on ethical issues occurs.

The concluding essay in Part One, coauthored with Raymond De Vries, "Bureaucracies of Mass Deception: Institutional Review Boards and the Ethics of Ethnographic Research," anticipates the concern for research ethics that characterizes the essays in Parts Two and Three. One of the major contributions of bioethics has been in the domain of research ethics. This contribution has a structural component, institutional review boards and the prospective ethical review of research, and an intellectual component, a burgeoning literature on questions of research ethics. This chapter explores the structural component and, in doing so, becomes part of that burgeoning literature. The essay explores how poorly the model of prospective review fits the procedures of ethnographic research, discusses social scientists' discontent and frustration with the bureaucratic and prospective review of research proposals, suggests some ways the entire system might be improved, and explores how, even if these improvements are adopted, the major ethical questions that come up while doing ethnography remain unexplored.

In the essays in Parts Two and Three, I try to look at the ethics of ethnography by raising questions about my own research. The essays in Part Two, "The Ethics of Ethnography: Genetic Counselors Revisited," look at the questions that fieldwork among genetic counselors raised for me. The first essay, "An Introduction to Ethnography," asks what difference it makes if one is asked into a setting by participants who want some help rather than, as is customary, worming one's way into a setting of one's choosing. The second essay, "A Twice-Told Tale of Witnessing," examines and critiques the procedures that I used in the fieldwork for my research on genetic counselors. The last essay in Part Two, "Irony, Ethnography, and Informed Consent," looks at the sense of betrayal the subjects of *All God's Mistakes* felt when they were given the opportunity to read the text. In the three chapters of Part Two, I seek to deepen our understanding both of the difficulties of informed consent and of the ways that being a research subject within a literate group may create unanticipated problems for group members.

Part Three revisits the fieldwork for *Forgive and Remember*. The first chapter, "The Field-Worker and the Surgeon," consists of my original reflections in the form of a fieldwork appendix. The next chapter, "An Ethnographer's Apology, a Bioethicist's Lament: The Surgeon and the Sociologist Revisited," is a retrospective reflection of how those things that I did to preserve the confidentiality and anonymity of my subjects served the organized interests of the institution that I studied more than they served any individual subjects. In particular, I discuss how a gender switch I made to disguise one of my subjects then made it impossible for me to discuss some of the more oppressive features of surgical residency. The chapter also describes what for me is one paradigm for the ethical dilemmas that ethnographers face: the conflict between equally important yet contradictory ethical values. When the first essay in Part Three first appeared, it was praised in many quarters as a model of candor; the second essay illustrates that it was a model of evasion as well. The concluding chapter in Part Three, "A Monument of Silence: On Not Giving Up Dr. Arthur's Ghost," describes the sense of betrayal that I felt when Pacific Hospital unblinded my original research in a fundraising appeal. It points out some of the difficulties that are involved when subjects are promised confidentiality and anonymity yet the researcher has little control over whether the promise will be kept.

The conclusion to this volume, "Professional Expertise and Moral Cowardice: Counterfeit Courage and the Noncombatant," asks once again the question "What would you do in my situation?" to consolidate the themes of this volume: the enduring relational tension between social science and ethics, the irreducible normative element in social theory, the always-present empirical element in ethics decision making, and the inherent confusions of the blurred academic genre empirical bioethics. The chapter sketches a role for the social science researcher engaged in the question of how "ethics" is defined and organized in various domains. My hope for that chapter, and for the entire volume, is that it contribute to the spirited discussion among the disciplines involved in "the collection of socially visible activities that we call bioethics" about the serious challenges that we as a community face in trying to make decisions on those Weberian questions of meaning for which neither the natural nor the social sciences can provide a satisfactory answer. My intent for this volume is to signal that healthy debate about these "human condition" questions that evoked such despair for Weber is likely to be more productive the thicker we allow it grow. I fear the thin gruel of smug answers or unquestioned formal procedures that are not open to revision. What needs to be balanced more than juggled as we struggle with the ethical dilemmas posed by our growing capacity to fiddle with ourselves, extend and enhance life, and forestall death but not prevent suffering are our need for solutions provided by professional experts and our ability to resist them in order to give others the autonomy that we would wish to exercise ourselves.

1

THE ETHNOGRAPHY OF ETHICS

ONE

Professional Ethicist Available

LOGICAL, SECULAR, FRIENDLY

> Problem resolution through ethics based decisionmaking. Professional ethicist provides practical supportive help with personal decisions. Logical, Secular, Friendly · PERSONALS ADVERTISEMENT[1]

Writing in 1919, Max Weber said:

Consider modern medicine, a practical technology which is highly developed scientifically. The general "presupposition" of the medical enterprise is stated trivially in the assertion that medical science has the task of maintaining life as such and of diminishing suffering as such to the greatest possible degree. Yet this is problematical. By his means the medical man preserves the life of the mortally ill man, even if the patient implores us to relieve him of life, even if his relatives to whom his life is worthless and to whom the costs of maintaining his worthless life grow unbearable, grant his redemption from suffering. . . . Yet the presuppositions of medicine, and the penal code, prevent the physician from relinquishing his therapeutic efforts. Whether life is worth while living and when—this question is not asked by medicine. Natural science gives us an answer to the question of what we must do if we wish to master life technically. It leaves quite aside, or assumes for its purposes, whether we should and do wish to master life technically and whether it makes ultimate sense to do so.[2]

Chapter 1 was originally published as "Professional Ethicist Available: Logical, Secular, Friendly," *Daedalus* 128, no. 4 (Fall 1999): 47–67.

What was true for Weber at the beginning of the century remains true for us postmoderns at its close—a technologically muscular medical science possesses on its own no wisdom about when and how it should be deployed. For Weber, the tragedy of modernity was the possibility of possessing the means to "master life" without any requisite wisdom about how to do so. But consider how much better equipped we are today to deal with Weber's "mortally ill man." If this man had any foresight, then he has a "living will" instructing his physicians how to manage the end of his life. If his physicians feel that his care is futile, they are empowered to discuss with the patient, if he or she is competent, or, if not, with the patient's family, what level of care the patient wishes. One possible outcome of these deliberations is a "Do Not Resuscitate" order entered in the patient's chart. If the family, patient, physicians, and nursing staff disagree about how to treat the last days of Weber's miserable man, then an "ethics consult" can be requested. Today, there is no shortage of procedures or moral experts able to speak to the questions on which science is silent—"whether we should and do wish to master life technically and whether it ultimately makes sense to do so."

How well these procedures accomplish their intended goals, how competently these experts provide satisfactory answers to those questions on which science is silent, are important questions. But to ask them this way—as if they were merely an exercise in policy assessment—implies that if these procedures or experts were found wanting, then some others are capable of producing "better" results. In a volume such as this on social science, ethics, and medicine, there is an almost irresistible temptation to make such an argument: namely, that the problems of bioethics are better handled using an approach that is more social scientific, that pays greater attention to culture and class, power and position, gender and ethnicity, than the standard bioethical explorations of how to manage problems like Weber's mortally ill man.

However, in this essay I wish to forgo the general pleasures afforded by preaching to the choir. As much as I might enjoy demonstrating from my own research how the trained sensitivities of the social scientist improve bioethical discourse, I think little new is gained by the exercise, it having been carried out so well so many times by so many others. Instead, I want to ask how it is that we are even in the position of having to demonstrate what should be obvious: that social science matters to bioethics. First, I want to explore how bioethics came to the dominant position it has today for discussing a whole range of questions about medical care. Second, I want to show what a surprising development is the emergence of bioethics as an applied discipline. In so doing, I want to ask how it is that social scientists who came to many of these issues before, or contemporaneously with, those philosophers who identify themselves as bioethicists now need to mount special pleas for our inclusion in, our relevance to, and our importance for the discourse of bioethics.

Looking Backwards

Now that there is a National Advisory Bioethics Commission, now that the Joint Commission on Accreditation of Healthcare Organizations mandates that hospitals need to have in place a mechanism for resolving ethical conflicts, now that numerous programs provide training that leads to certificates and degrees in bioethics, now that the graduates of these programs seek employment as "clinical ethicists," now that professional organizations and journals in bioethics have proliferated, now that a task force assembled under the aegis of the major professional societies in bioethics has issued a "consensus statement" on standards for "clinical ethics" practice and its practitioners, and now that over fifty academic medical centers have departments of or centers for bioethics, it is fairly simple to tell a "Whiggish" history of bioethics—one that makes not only its structural position but also its current intellectual configurations appear as both inevitable and desirable.

This history (which actually has more the structure of an "origins myth") is certainly familiar by now. Over the last thirty or so years, bioethics has been a response to a sense of crisis within the everyday organization of medicine. Some of that crisis was generated internally. Reports like Raymond Duff and Angus Campbell's classic 1973 *New England Journal of Medicine* article on the withdrawal of life support for severely compromised neonates after consultation with parents at Yale–New Haven Hospital took private clinical troubles and made them a public issue for the profession.[3] The crusading dimension to Duff and Campbell's discussion, the if-this-be-treason-make-the-most-of-it rhetoric, is hard to overlook:

> What are the legal implications of actions like those described in this paper? . . . Perhaps more than anything else, the public and professional silence on a major social taboo and some common practices has been broken further. That seems appropriate, for out of the ensuing dialogue perhaps better choices for patients and their families can be made. If working out these dilemmas in ways such as we suggest is in violation of the law, we believe the law should be changed.[4]

Duff and Campbell's article discussed neonatal intensive care, a rather recent and, at that time, still primitive technological development; but their essay spoke as well to all those other clinical arenas within medicine that had likewise expanded technologically, creating tensions for those now managing Weber's hypothetical "mortally ill man" that Weber himself could never have imagined. What for Weber had been problematic at a theoretical level given medicine's limited capacities in the early years of the twentieth century had now become empirically and emotionally difficult at the everyday level.

A second internalist critique appeared in the normally august pages of the *New England Journal of Medicine* when Henry Beecher published an exposé of physicians' conduct of scientific research.[5] Deliberate deception, a lack of a minimal concern with consent, sloppily designed trials unlikely to yield useful information, and overly risky protocols were among the faults that concerned Beecher. Like his colleagues at Yale, the Harvard physician had an innate faith that if problems became public, then they would be addressed. As David Rothman claims in his informative account of both the extent of and the limits to Beecher's whistle-blowing:

> He noted with more rhetorical flourish than evidence or accuracy that the "thoughtlessness and carelessness [of the researchers with unethical protocols], not a willful disregard of the patient's rights, account for most of the cases encountered." Armed with such a formulation, he comfortably asserted that "calling attention . . . will help to correct the abuses present." He maintained such an old-fashioned faith in the integrity of the individual researcher that, after weighing all the alternatives, he concluded: "The more reliable safeguard [is] provided by the presence of an intelligent, informed, conscientious, compassionate, responsible investigator."[6]

There is something particularly American about this melioristic faith that open communication leads to solutions. There is little to no recognition by the authors of either article that problems may be intractable; values, discordant; goals, divergent; and decisions (or resolutions), difficult.

The very same criticisms that were made inside medicine were also made outside of it. The end-of-life questions asked in the *New England Journal of Medicine* by Duff and Campbell were also posed by Elisabeth Kubler-Ross in her trade publication *On Death and Dying*.[7] The University of Chicago psychiatrist criticized medical practice for its emphasis on managing dying through a dehumanizing technological regime that ignored death's spiritual and emotional dimensions:

> Maybe this question has to be raised: Are we becoming less human or more human? Though this book is in no way meant to be judgmental, it is clear that whatever the answer may be, the patient is suffering more—not physically, perhaps, but emotionally. And his needs have not changed over the centuries, only our ability to gratify them.[8]

Here Kubler-Ross is exhibiting some of the denial that she claims is part of the first stage in adapting to a terminal diagnosis. It is hard to read *On Death and Dying* without being impressed by how judgmental it is. One of these judgments is that there is an emotionally correct way to die that crosses generations, classes, and cultural groupings. While Kubler-Ross is a physician, it is important for our purposes to note that she makes her critique largely outside professional domains and her appeals are directed as much at patients and families, who should demand better, as at health professionals, who should know better. Her account, in fact, emphasizes the obstacles medical staff placed in front of her work.

> As described earlier, the hospital staff responded with great resistance, at times overt hostility, to our seminar. At the beginning, it was almost impossible to get permission from the attending staff to interview one of their patients. Residents were more difficult to approach than interns, the latter more resistant than externs or medical students. It appeared the more training a physician had, the less he was ready to become involved in this type of work.[9]

A few years after the public discussion on the significance of the fact that public discussion of death and dying was no longer taboo, which Kubler-Ross's work in part fueled, a series of media-intensive "right to die" cases emerged, the most important of which was that of Karen Anne Quinlan. Besides the enormous amount of coverage and, hence, collective awareness of ethical dilemmas in modern medicine the case generated, two features of it are worth noting here. First, this was not a conflict that could be resolved within the normal doctor-patient relationship. Even if Karen Anne's physicians agreed with her parents' decision to disconnect her respirator, they felt the need for legal protection and approval before embarking on this course. The structure of the legal process made Karen Anne Quinlan's parents and her physicians adversaries, which clearly showed that both the nature and the pace of this process rendered it inadequate for resolving conflict in instant cases. A considerable amount of the commentary on the case as it unfolded centered on why we are, as a collectivity, trying to solve this problem in this way. Second, this structural impasse did not escape the New Jersey Supreme Court, which, while seeing the right to die as a privacy issue, nonetheless recommended that hospitals use ethics committees to resolve such problems and thereby keep them out of the courts. Such a policy, when followed, makes private decisions more public and requires individuals willing to claim expertise in ethical decision making. It assumes as well that such expertise will serve to silence social conflict. And, to the social scientist, this expectation—that an ethics process internalized within the hospital will reduce conflict—may be the feature of clinical ethics most worth exploring.

As with death and dying, in the domain of research ethics much of the criticism made within medicine was made from outside of medicine. Two research projects in particular received considerable media attention. Both involved the exploitation of vulnerable populations in federally sponsored research. The first was the infamous Tuskegee Syphilis Study. This "natural history" of untreated syphilis in black males involved researchers actively preventing subjects who were poor black sharecroppers from receiving medical treatments. The subjects were never informed that they were in a research project that forbade treatment. The second project involved the injecting of retarded children at Willowbrook, a residential treatment center, with Hepatitis B in order to test a vaccine. As in Tuskegee, consent was forgone. These research abuses were not discovered by the medical profession. Rather, the fact that they were uncovered by journalists and were then the subject of legislative hearings was taken as evidence of the failure of internal reform. Those outside of medicine confronting these abuses felt, unlike Beecher, that if these ethical problems of medicine were to be faced, it would be because of pressure and resources brought from the outside. Moreover, and this seems odd in today's antiregulatory atmosphere, such outside scrutiny fit the temper of the times. There was something like a national consensus that institutional domains, such as medical practice and research, could be made more accountable only through a greater surveillance of their activities. In this spirit, medicine was one of many institutional domains subject to the antiseptic and disinfectant effects of the sunshine of public surveillance.

And, in a manner of speaking, the problems of deceitful research were faced from the outside. A National Commission for the Protection of Human

Subjects of Biomedical and Behavioral Research was formed, which promulgated regulations after holding hearings and deliberations. These regulations, when adopted, required that all institutions receiving federal funds have institutional review boards in place to monitor research protocols for the adequacy of consent procedures and of risk-benefit ratios. The National Commission was followed in a few years' time by a President's Commission for the Study of Ethical Problems in Medicine and Biomedical and Behavioral Research. Whatever else may be said of the work of the President's Commission, and the National Commission before it, at a very minimum each legitimated public discourse by nonmedical experts on problematic areas of medical practice and research. The doctor-patient relationship was now very much a public concern. The documents that the President's Commission produced serve either as informal national practice guidelines or, less grandly, as a baseline for public debate and discussion. The most recent legitimating event for bioethics has been the appointment of a permanent National Bioethics Advisory Commission. What is significant here, and in each of the preceding moves, is the public approval given to the idea that what is wrong with health care is somehow connected to ethics and that such problems are best fixed by ethicists. The entire nature of the debate inside and outside the profession has acted either to squeeze other definitions of the problems outside the arena of discourse or to force other critics to frame their critiques in terms set by bioethics and bioethicists.

Looking Forward

As I have stated, this brief sketch of the growing dominance of bioethics is decidedly Whiggish—it thinks backwards about a complex chain of events and selects for emphasis only those that make the current state of affairs seem natural, inevitable, and desirable. Of course, to tell the story this way is a distortion; more than that, it obscures first what kind of change bioethics represents and, second, how peculiar a development is the emergence of bioethics, especially as a clinical specialty.

The typical account of bioethics coming to its present position in the medical center celebrates its "transformational" or "revolutionary" impact on medical practice. The claim is often advanced that with its emphasis on patient autonomy, bioethics played a large role in overturning a regime of physician paternalism and replacing it with one that was patient centered. Such a claim overstates how much of a challenge bioethics posed to medicine. Although at certain points the bioethicist's critique seems to be a broad indictment of medical practice, it is actually quite limited. For the bioethicist, the problem is not one of structural arrangements, the distribution of power, privilege, and authority, or the culture of medicine itself—all of which call for the expertise of the social scientist and suggest the need for more radical, structural change than bioethics has wrought. The problems of medical practice, as defined by bioethicists, are ones of values in a relationship. Place the right values in the doctor-patient relationship and the problems disappear. From the perspective of bioethics, it was as if everything was right with the way medicine was practiced except for what was said and how it was said in certain very exceptional circumstances. Those exceptional circumstances, the problematic beginnings and endings of life, were precisely those areas where Weber had noted that science was silent, areas where the presuppositions of medicine as science prevented the questioning of effort. Beyond that, they were areas where new technological capacities made those issues appear somehow discontinuous with their prior incarnations as "human condition problems," which medical professionals have always had to face.

If one assumption of bioethics is that the problems of medicine are located at the level of the individual doctor-patient relationship and consist of the inappropriate values operating within that relationship, then a second assumption is that bioethicists can fix or ameliorate the problem by correctly analyzing that values problem. Where this idea comes from, whether philosophers actively sold it to physicians, or whether physicians on their own promoted it, is not so critical to determine here. Rather, what is worthy of our attention is how naive the idea that ethical analysis leads effectively to ethical practice seems when stated plainly. After all, there are not many areas where we equate theoretical and practical wisdom. We have cultural myths about lawyers dying intestate, cobblers' children running around unshod, and mental-health professionals whose entire being screams for a few effective therapeutic interventions. Further, the idea that moral theory can be used to solve practical problems cuts against so many beliefs prevalent in the medical, academic, or larger political culture that we might wonder about its centrality to the bioethics enterprise. What I want to emphasize here is how odd was the idea that bioethics through moral philosophy or ethical theory had something concrete to offer the clinician.

To do that, I want to recapture a sense of the medical and academic environment as I thought it existed the first time I heard the word *bioethics*, on the first occasion I heard someone introduced as a bioethicist. The time was the spring of 1974; the occasion was a symposium on Ethics, the Law, and Abortion at the University of Chicago Law School; and the speaker was

Daniel Callahan, who headed up an organization I had until that moment never heard of—The Hastings Center of something or other (I did not catch at the time the longer, proper description of the organization, and I was certainly unaware that my private trouble correctly recalling that longer title was to become something of a public issue). At the time, I was a graduate student doing fieldwork in surgery—I certainly would not have identified myself as a medical sociologist. In fact, I am certain that I did not yet realize that sociologists were categorized by their research interests or methods. Looking back, I wonder now what attracted me to the symposium. The University of Chicago had an unquestionably rich schedule of intellectually stimulating gatherings, but I was in the last lap of my graduate work and not easily coaxed away from my tasks. But there I was.

I do not remember much of Callahan's talk save for his brief definition of bioethics—the application of ethical theory to the dilemmas raised by the practice of modern medicine, especially those problems created by the application of new technologies—and my reaction, which was swift and savage, balanced somewhere between hostility and incredulity. If I had ever heard a nonstarter of an idea, this was it. This reaction was not just the hostility to philosophical speculation that had been part of my sociological training; this was more than the standard injunction to concentrate on what is and avoid speculation about what ought to be, although the repetition of that part of a social scientist's credo must have exercised some impact. No, this reaction was based on my understanding of medical culture from the scant fieldwork that I had already conducted. The reaction was also surprising to me in that my limited observations of medicine suggested that ethical questions did indeed need to be aired.

What I had learned living among surgeons was that to characterize an issue as "ethical" signaled a number of things. First, issues that were "ethical" were seen as issues that were not resolvable. There was no gold standard against which to measure responses, against which to credit some as correct and dismiss others as wrong. The corollary of this was that ethical issues could be debated forever with no resolution. Since surgery had an ethic of action, such debate was seen as a waste of everyone's time. My fieldwork was done in an academic setting, in a prestigious training program, as a visible observer scribbling into a small notebook, so, from time to time, attending surgeons might display their ethical reasoning either because they had been asked to, because they thought it didactically necessary, or because they cared what the observer thought of them. But the general feeling was that ethical discussion wasted time, effort, and energy—it stole time from caring for patients, reading journals, dictating discharge summaries, or practicing knot tying. Those students who pressed ethical questions were often asked sarcastically if they wanted to be internists or surgeons. A correlate of this was that whenever I raised ethical issues in my field notes or discussions with my principal adviser, he would ask me with more than a little irritation if I were writing a dissertation or preparing for the rabbinate. So, however aware I was that ethical questions needed a fuller discussion than they were receiving, I was also aware of a general hostility toward such questions.

In general, cases that raised ethical questions were both abundant and rarely discussed. For example, during the eighteen months of my fieldwork, a young black male who had lost all but four inches of his bowel to a gunshot wound and an incompetent resident, who was on call the night this patient was rolled in, was kept alive, while an attending tried to work out in his lab some of the problems that inhibited successful bowel transplants. The patient had no idea what was going on. I never once heard the ethical dimensions of the case discussed by the entire group during rounds or any other conference; my notes only record two times when residents or students mentioned the ethical dimensions of the case and then just barely: "I wouldn't want to be kept alive like that." This is not to say that the case was not discussed, because it was, but always from a very narrow, technical point of view: the problems of alimentation, the inevitability of rejection reactions, the reasons the four other attempted bowel transplants to date had so decisively failed, the promising new leads in the laboratory. Nor is it to say that the attending in question did not consider the "ethics" of the case. I am certain that he did—he was an unusually thoughtful and reflective person—he simply did not "share" his thoughts with the group. And this lack of sharing was itself important: it indexed a primary belief about ethics. With authority went responsibility—ethics were personal. Attendings had an unquestioned and, at the time I did my observations, socially unquestionable decision-making authority. There were decisions that "only an attending could make." Little was gained by public debate of such situations. Young apprentice surgeons were taught that there were tough ethical decisions, that these were personal, that they need not be discussed or reflected upon in an open forum, and that making such decisions was a prerogative of rank. They were in training so that when their time came they would not flinch before this burden. A suggestion or proposal that a patient or a nurse might question a surgeon's handling of a case or that they had the capacity to have that handling reviewed by an ethics consultant or an ethics committee was Swiftian in its preposterous implausibility.

Now I suppose that since I knew that surgery was not the entire world of academic medicine, that there were strong cultural differences between surgery and internal medicine, and that in internal medicine there was a higher tolerance for both discussion and "theoretical" issues, I should not have been so quick to dismiss bioethics as a doomed enterprise. But I had noticed that when surgeons and internists disagreed about patient care, those disputes were resolved by figuring out whose patient it was. Both surgeons and internists seemed to agree that ethical decisions were reserved for the physician in charge. Further, I had, by that time, attended a few joint internal medicine-general surgery conferences on the management of the terminal patient. From the sentiments expressed in those meetings, I could see no differences in the decision-making prerogatives given to the physician in charge. I could not help but notice that there was less hierarchy in internal medicine. This meant that residents in internal medicine had to arrive at their own personal philosophy or ethics of care much sooner than residents in surgery, who were often shielded from such issues as they perfected their technical skills. Looking back, what I now see, but did not realize at the time, is that residents in internal medicine, who were left so alone with such weighty questions so early in their careers, would find the help bioethicists promised attractive. Certainly, a major recurring theme of the first-hand narratives of physicians who trained during this time period is that the steady hand and cool reason of a more seasoned authority is absent.[10] The texts fairly scream with rage at how much the physician in training has been abandoned, at how little guidance is provided for such complex human-condition questions.

There were two other reasons why I thought, while listening to Callahan, that medicine was not likely to find bioethics attractive. First, I did not observe that physicians were receptive to the collateral expertise of other professionals. Callahan was defining a substantive domain in which philosophers could provide physicians with help. I could not help but notice that the physicians I was observing had some trouble asking for help with ethical or, for that matter, any other sorts of problems. It was a difficult enough matter to get the surgeons to consult already established services appropriately rather than ignore them. Medical social workers were consulted only when there were obvious discharge problems. Psychiatric liaison was seen as a distasteful last resort, often used when the importunings of nurses made it impossible to stall any longer. The input of nurses was very rarely sought; when offered unsolicited, it was listened to more as a tactic of keeping social peace than because it promised to be useful. And while all this may seem either to be exaggerated or to be just an indicator of surgical boorishness, I thought about it differently. If those with training, clinical experience, and an established place in the hospital hierarchy were not taken seriously, then I did not see how it was possible that outsiders, namely, bioethicists, would establish a foothold. Here, what I missed was the role physicians with an interest in medical ethics would play in sponsoring the concerns of bioethics and bioethicists.

Next, there was something about the "values talk" of bioethicists that I thought would not play well in medical domains. The ethical problems that I had observed—that is to say, those problems that were openly recognized and categorized as ethical (there were ethical problems aplenty that never got so labeled and were, as a consequence, never viewed through the lens of ethics)—cried out for immediate solutions. These cases were, as I viewed them as a fieldworker, mired in contextual details often so different from case to case that I could not imagine any set of values or principles so flexible that they would permit generalization across cases. I thought, quite wrongly, that whatever an approach grounded in ethics had to offer, it would be so abstract that physicians seeking guidance would only experience frustration. After all, I could not help but notice how relentlessly empirical physicians were—rigorous positivists, they scorned nothing so much as data that were "anecdotal" or explanations that were "speculative." Again I was wrong and it is easy to identify why. I did not appreciate how compatible the thin sociological description of the medical case was with the thin sociological description of the philosophical one. In each case, the thinness served a purpose: the physician was able to concentrate on pathophysiology; the philosopher, on principles. Neither needed to deal with the variety of ways in which the social context muddies the waters. In addition, I did not appreciate how the conceptual flexibility of the philosopher's principles served the physician seeking legitimation for a course of action. Action and principles needed only be described in ways that emphasized their fit. The more general the principle, the easier the task. So what I saw initially as burdens to the adoption of bioethics turned out, on closer inspection, to be benefits.

Those were the obstacles that occurred to me at the time, and they seemed sufficient to stop any further exploration. I had good reasons for expecting bioethics to fail to take root in the academic medical center. Had I the need to find additional reasons to predict the failure of the "bioethics project," I would not have needed to look very far. Three additional disabling factors suggest themselves. First, the role being proposed for bioethics and bioethicists was one that was increasingly out of favor among academic moral philosophers. After all, a major selling point of bioethics within the medical center was the ability of moral philosophers to provide a problem-solving methodology for the vexing day-to-day troubles of modern medicine (of course, not all those involved in bioethics promised this). The dominant approach, in the field's dominant text, principlism, seemed to offer a short-cut for reasoning through some difficult troubles.[11] Principlism, which was not without its critics, is alluring because it is not only comprehensible but appears easy to apply and, thus, removes from ethical questions the earlier stigma conferred by their being unresolvable. But it was just this claim that ethical theory had direct problem-solving capabilities that was being widely rejected within academic philosophy.[12]

This schism between the applied philosophers in the medical center and the theoreticians of the academy had, however, little impact on the recruits to or the development of bioethics. One reason is that medical centers had resources at their disposal that philosophy departments did not. Bioethics programs, institutes, and centers were started within medical centers, and some journals were underwritten there. Whatever academic philosophers thought of all this, whether they thought that the ethics that medicine had saved the life of was worth saving,[13] mattered little in the face of the resources medical centers commanded. If academic philosophers disapproved, then bioethics programs in medical centers would train the personnel needed as ethicists. If the prestigious journals in philosophy were uninterested in the applied questions on which bioethicists wrote, then there were new outlets for such writing aplenty. All of this means that bioethics developed within the institutional structure and with the institutional resources of academic medicine, and this undoubtedly influenced its critical thrust. At the same time, the fact that its oldest and best-known institution, The Hastings Center, was free standing helped sustain an illusion of the field's independence. It meant as well that this branch of applied ethics could safely ignore, or dismiss as sour grapes, the criticisms of colleagues in academic departments.

Not only was the field of bioethics with the bioethicist in the role of clinical ethicist contrary to currents within academic philosophy departments, but the framework of principlism that guided so many of the day-to-day applications of bioethics was itself out of step with trends in the surrounding culture. Advocates of principlism suggest that the application of four values—autonomy, beneficence, nonmaleficence, and justice—is sufficient to resolve ethical problems as they arise in the clinic. This is not the place to rehearse the criticisms of principlism, the defense of those criticisms, the revisions of the original formulations, or the modifications that allowed principlism to gear into the world as a guide to action. Here, I want simply to call attention to leading assumptions of principlism: namely, that the individual is the proper measure of all things ethical, that tools for measurement transcend culture, and that there is a single, correct solution for each ethical problem, which is largely independent of person, place, or time. At the time that this ethical universalism is gaining ascendance in the world of medicine, it is being rejected in virtually every other sphere of society. In academia, cultural relativism had made the assertion of a single ethical standard applied across cultures highly problematic. In the public arena of political culture, the spirit of cultural pluralism made the assertion of such a single standard not only unfashionable but also a badge of great insensitivity. The fact that bioethics embraced principlism and that this embrace took root in such a complex community as the modern medical center is peculiar, to say the least. Of course, the very nature of principlism gave it a curious dual aspect. On the one hand, the four principles seemed to provide something like a moral methodology for public discussion of ethical issues. John Evans has even suggested that principlism functions in ethics much as double-entry bookkeeping does in accounting: it makes commensurable what was formerly incommensurable.[14] On the other hand, despite the seemingly privileged place of autonomy, the fact that principlism allows the four principles to be combined and deployed in any configuration allows a wide range of cultural preferences legitimation under its aegis.[15] Principlism has then the seeming advantage of being both authoritative and sensitive to cultural difference.

Finally, bioethics had to struggle against a resistance to rule by experts in American society. The questions that advocates for bioethics felt most comfortable addressing were almost exclusively questions of "bedside ethics." However, here one might ask why the paternalistic judgment of one expert should be replaced by that of another. Further, the basis of granting legitimacy to the physician was grounded in a long-standing cultural logic. This was not so for the moral authority of the bioethicist, which was being created on the spot. The fact that bioethicists spoke of what they were doing as restoring power to patients obscured the power they needed to create for themselves to accomplish this task. It also obscured how much patients actually desired this decision-making power now conferred upon them. It is worth noting in this light how rarely the resources for a more muscular assertion of patient autonomy are utilized.

A Temporizing Conclusion in the Present

I have tried to sketch how bioethics ascended to its current dominant position and to give a sense of the many cultural obstacles it had to overcome in doing so. I probably have not conveyed as clearly as I might how, all of the above notwithstanding, bioethics was a response to deeply felt needs within both the medical community and the larger society. In concluding, I want to turn to the task that I eschewed at the beginning of the essay—defining where social science might fit into the bioethics project. But the prolix prologue to what will be a spare set of conclusions is in some sense a demonstration of the major role that the social sciences play within bioethics: the provision of context, the gentle insistence that principles are attached to persons, and the constant reminder that those persons have interests, a history, and a culture. Three examples will suffice to sketch the role for the social sciences that I have in mind, to show the difference that richer contextual accounts make.

First, now that bioethics has some institutional anchorage and cultural legitimacy, a number of histories of bioethics have emerged. These accounts are somewhat triumphalist in tone, seeing bioethics as a victory of patients over medical authority. These histories associate the rise and ultimate success of bioethics with the success of rights-based movements more generally. The account of bioethics' rise to prominence offered here tempers this triumphalism by showing how limited was the challenge presented to organized medicine. Had space permitted a fuller discussion, I would have shown that bioethics was a contemporaneous alternative to a more forceful challenge to medicine spearheaded by consumer and patient activists. This later challenge was more confrontational in tone, more insistent on structural change, and more focused on the politics of health care than was the bioethics movement. By assimilating bioethics, organized medicine was able to defang this other, broader challenge. Even without a full discussion of this alternative to bioethics, my account stresses the interests that were involved in bioethics coming to the fore and emphasizes the fit of bioethics with academic medicine. This is not to say that bioethicists' claims that they have provided patients a greater voice in determining their own affairs are incorrect. It does provide data, however, to allow us to question whether those changes are as dramatic as their promoters would have us believe. Also, by pointing out how bioethics' triumph is related to how limited was its challenge to organized medical interests, we are also in a position to understand why bioethicists have not raised a number of political issues that also can be defined as ethical questions: the presence of so many millions of Americans without health insurance, the multiple ways the production pressures of managed care undercut the possibilities of the doctor-patient relationship that bioethics celebrates, the inequalities in health status between rich and poor, or the replacement of professional values with corporate ones.

Second, we social scientists provide just the kind of context bioethicists so often obscure when we produce ethnographies of medical settings that describe as thickly as possible how ethical problems are ignored, unattended, recognized, managed, and resolved in medical settings. There are good recent examples in which ethical problems in the medical workplace are a focus of the analysis.[16] But the goal is not to show how these problems are properly or improperly resolved. Rather, the focus is on how the problems are structured. These examples show first how problems in the workplace of the hospital come to be seen as ethical, and then what this labeling accomplishes in terms of conflict management. In each work, problems that an earlier period would have addressed as problems in the organization of work, the division of labor and responsibility, and the structure of authority are now labeled as ethical. This labeling allows power differentials between the ranks of doctors, nurses, and patients to be effaced. It also allows a hearing for the nurses' and patients' perspectives on what should be done, which would not happen unless the problems were understood as "ethical"—a domain that bioethicists assume operates outside of the social structure. By bringing the context of dispute into the bioethics discourse, social scientists deepen our understanding of the ethical conflict and question the assumption that the right thinking with the right values will suffice to silence the conflict.

In a very real way, if ethnographies of medical settings are properly done, they may very well cut against the objectives of bioethicists. There may be a built-in incompatibility between bioethical and sociological inquiry, and heightening this tension rather than attempting to deny it may very well be a useful contribution of the social scientist to bioethics. The purpose of bioethical inquiry, I assume, is to clarify which principles should guide action when decision is difficult. In bioethics, descriptions of motives, intents, and purposes need to be fairly one-dimensional or the balancing of values gets too complex for application. The goal of social science, especially as practiced by ethnographers (again, this is my assumption), is to show how actors shape and trim their actions to fit their principles and how these same actors shape and trim their values and principles to fit their actions. Where bioethicists seek clarity, social scientists look for ambiguity and complexity. Social scientists are eager to show that our subjects are not slavish followers of rules, that they are not in principle or action "judgmental dopes,"[17] but that they have great flexibility in deciding which rules to apply and when to apply them. If one thinks about this, this is a message at odds with the goals of bioethical analysis: identify a situation correctly and decide what principles apply, and ethical behavior will follow. These premises are implicitly challenged by ethnographic accounts. Clarity about values for the social scientist is very seldom a reassurance that any specific behavior will occur in the next instant. Social scientists are more sensitive than bioethicists to the well-known lag between values and behaviors. A contribution that social scientists can make and remake to bioethics is a close inspection of the fit between what we do and what we say we are doing—our actions and our intentions.

Finally, social scientists can contribute to bioethics by studying this discipline. When sociologists are invited into bioethics, aid is sought for pre-identified problems. We social scientists are invited to join the team. Flattering as this invitation is, social science may aid bioethics more by declining the offer. (This, I realize, may read somewhat disingenuously; it is being written, after all, by someone with a faculty appointment in a Center for Bioethics. But, in my own defense, let me say that ethnographers have long realized that the proper balance of nearness and distance is difficult to achieve.) Bioethicist is a new role, and we know very little of how it works in the everyday medical contexts of its use. What do bioethicists do? For whom? Under what conditions? We need to contextualize bioethics itself and see it as an object of study. We have done precious little of this. And plainly we need to do more. How are bioethicists trained? How do those in the field define their domain of responsibility? How is orthodoxy established? How is dissent managed? These are beginning questions. In asking them, we need to ask broader questions as well. How is moral authority constructed and legitimated in the case of bioethicists? How is the role and moral authority attached to it connected to an increased concern for ethics in other societal domains? Social scientists have contributed and will continue to contribute to our understanding of many of the substantive problems in the domain of bioethics. These contributions, however, should not blind us to the contribution we have yet to make: the description and analysis of the everyday work of people in the new social role we now call bioethicist.

Notes

1. Personals advertisement, *The Nation*, 13 June 1994.
2. Max Weber, "Science as a Vocation" (1919, 1922) in H. H. Gerth and C. Wright Mills, eds., *From Max Weber: Essays in Sociology* (New York: Oxford University Press, 1946), 144.
3. Raymond Duff and Angus Campbell, "Moral and Ethical Dilemmas in the Special Care Nursery," *New England Journal of Medicine* 289 (1973): 890–94.
4. Ibid., 894.

5. Henry Beecher, "Ethics in Clinical Research," *New England Journal of Medicine* 274 (1966): 1354–60.

6. David J. Rothman, *Strangers at the Bedside: A History of How Law and Bioethics Transformed Medical Decision Making* (New York: Basic Books, 1991), 83–84.

7. Elisabeth Kubler-Ross, *On Death and Dying* (New York; Macmillan, 1969).

8. Ibid., 10.

9. Ibid., 245.

10. Samuel Shem, *The House of God* (New York: Dell, 1979); Charles LeBaron, *Gentle Vengeance: An Account of the First Year at Harvard Medical School* (New York: R. Marek, 1981); and Kenneth Klein, *Getting Better: A Medical Student's Story* (Boston and Toronto: Little, Brown, and Co., 1981).

11. Tom L. Beauchamp and James F. Childress, *Principles of Biomedical Ethics* (New York and Oxford: Oxford University Press, 1979).

12. Bernard Williams, *Moral Luck* (Cambridge and New York: Cambridge University Press, 1981); Stuart Hampshire, *Morality and Conflict* (Cambridge, Mass.: Harvard University Press, 1983); Alasdair C. MacIntyre, *After Virtue: A Study in Moral Theory* (Notre Dame, Ind.: University of Notre Dame Press, 1981); and Michele M. Moody-Adams, *Fieldwork in Familiar Places: Morality, Culture, and Philosophy* (Cambridge, Mass.: Harvard University Press, 1997).

13. Steven Toulmin, "How Medicine Saved the Life of Ethics," *Perspectives in Biology and Medicine* 25 (1982): 736–50.

14. John Evans, "Max Weber Meets the Belmont Report: Toward a Sociological Account of Principlism," paper presented at "The Conference on the 20th Anniversary of the Belmont Report: Past and Future Directions," University of Virginia, Charlottesville, Va., April 1999.

15. Paul Wolpe, "The Triumph of Autonomy in American Bioethics: A Sociological View," in Raymond DeVries and Janardan Subedi, eds., *Bioethics and Society: Constructing the Ethical Enterprise* (Upper Saddle River, N.J.: Prentice Hall, 1998).

16. These include Renee R. Anspach, *Deciding Who Lives: Fateful Choices in the Intensive Care Nursery* (Berkeley: University of California Press, 1993); Charles L. Bosk, *All God's Mistakes: Genetic Counseling in a Pediatric Hospital* (Chicago: University of Chicago Press, 1992); Daniel F. Chambliss, *Beyond Caring: Hospitals, Nurses, and the Social Organization of Ethics* (Chicago: University of Chicago Press, 1996); Renée C. Fox and Judith P. Swazey, *Spare Parts: Organ Replacement in American Society* (New York: Oxford University Press, 1992); Carol A. Heimer and Lisa R. Staffen, *For the Sake of the Children: The Social Organization of Responsibility in the Hospital and Home* (Chicago: University of Chicago Press, 1998); and Robert Zussman, *Intensive Care: Medical Ethics and the Medical Profession* (Chicago: University of Chicago Press, 1992).

17. Harold Garfinkel, *Studies in Ethnomethodology* (Englewood Cliffs, N.J.: Prentice-Hall, 1967).

TWO

The Licensing and Certification of Ethics Consultants

WHAT PART OF "NO!" WAS SO HARD TO UNDERSTAND?

In *Core Competencies for Health Care Ethics Consultation,* the Task Force on Standards for Bioethics Consultation (of which I was a member) had this to say about certification:

> *Voluntary Guidelines.* The Task Force unanimously recommends that the content of this report be used as voluntary guidelines. Whether these guidelines are adopted by health care organizations or education and training programs should be based on an informed discussion of the report's merits. The Task Force:
>
> · Does not wish certifying or accrediting bodies to mandate any portion of its report
> · Believes that certification of individuals or groups to do ethics consultation is, at best, premature
> · Does not intend for its report [to be] used to establish a legal national standard for competence to do ethical consultation for the reasons indicated below.[1]

Chapter 2 was originally published as "The Licensing and Certification of Ethics Consultants: What Part of 'No!' Was so Hard to Understand?" in *Doing Ethics Consultation,* ed. Mark P. Aulisio, Robert M. Arnold, and Stuart A. Youngner. (Baltimore: Johns Hopkins University Press, 2003), 147–63.

"The reasons indicated below," the sparse commentary on the summary judgment, included the possible displacement of providers and patients as "the primary decision makers at the bedside"; the potential for authoritarian approaches to ethical decision making to emerge; the implicit endorsement of the mistaken proposition that certified individuals have some special standing to engage in decision making; the undermining of disciplinary diversity within bioethics; the establishment of a substantive ethical orthodoxy that brooks no dissent; the lack of an available and reliable measure of competence; the inability of the task force to imagine such a measure; and the raft of undesired economic, political, and pragmatic consequences that would float on any administrative scheme for implementing certification. The task force, then, spends a paragraph explaining that all the problems created by certifying individuals apply to the accreditation of committees as well.[2]

The penultimate paragraph of the report explains the use of the phrase "at this time" in the sentence, "Thus, at this time, the Task Force recommends that its report be used only as voluntary guidelines."[3] The explanation is simple. "At this time" does not contemplate some later time just over the horizon when it is appropriate to make these guidelines mandatory. Rather, "at this time" is what linguists call a "hedge" term. The task force did not think that mandatory guidelines were a good idea at the time of the report's submission. The task force could not imagine that set of conditions under which mandatory guidelines would become appropriate. Yet, when the task force submitted the report, it wanted to acknowledge that, "but, of course, we may be wrong about this,"[4] so it hedged with an "at this time."

I have quoted so fully from the conclusion of the report for two reasons. First, some of the commentators on the report have discounted its plain language and insist on reading it as an opening salvo in an ongoing struggle for professional accreditation. Among these commentators are some who see the sole purpose of the task force as furthering the professionalization of bioethics. For these commentators, the fact of the task force itself was a step toward this goal. The report, with its inevitable talk of standards and guidelines, inches us along this road. From guidelines it is a short stroll to certification. At the end of the journey, bioethicists, who once celebrated their distance from the medical model and saw their work as restoring autonomy to patients and leveling the playing field for medical action, will have created a professional presence that parallels the one they once sought to displace. There are those who might even argue, task force or not, certification or not, that much of this professional cooptation of bioethics, much of this blunting of any critical thrust, has not only occurred but also had a certain inevitability about it, given the conditions under which bioethicists are routinely employed.[5] After all, as the medical historian Charles Rosenberg remarked, "Ours is a health-care system, moreover, that has consistently demonstrated the ability to incorporate the critically and morally oppositional and make it an aspect of the system."[6]

The other reason I have quoted so fully from the conclusions of the report is that I have been assigned the task of commenting on what comes after the conclusion. What does the future hold? Is certification desirable? Inevitable? Are the critics of the report right to be so skeptical of how voluntary the guidelines are intended to be? Is bioethics consultation a professional activity? If so, does that make consultants professionals? If so, what standards of accountability apply to their actions? Who enforces those standards? It is, of course, much easier to generate a cascade of questions than to formulate a few coherent answers. In this chapter, rather than lay out an answer to the question of what the future holds for bioethics consultation and bioethics consultants, I shall lay out an approach for thinking about the question. That approach focuses on two different sociological questions. Who is a professional? And how is accountability for action achieved?

Who is a Professional?

At some level, controversy over whether the ASBH report is a step toward professionalizing ethics consultation services is most peculiar. After all, whoever provides the service, be it a physician, nurse, social worker, chaplain, psychologist, attorney, or philosopher, is a professional in some other domain. The organization in which the service is being provided is itself one that is thoroughly professionalized. So what is this debate about? How is it that ethics consultants are professionals in all their actions, save for ethics consulting? Beyond that, we need to ask, how does certifying or denying professional status to the ethics consultant affect the service being provided? What is at stake here? Why is this a label that some seek and others reject?

One way to assess this, to assess what difference it makes whether ethical consultants are considered professionals providing an expert service, is to look carefully at the social implications of work and workers being designated "professional." There are within sociology two competing perspectives on the meaning of *professional* that are germane here. Why the professionalization of ethics consulting services is so disturbing to so many becomes clear when the implications of these sociological perspectives are drawn out. In this exercise, it is important to keep in mind that although the perspectives compete within sociology, nonsociologists have no necessity to view the perspectives as alternative ways of explaining the same empirical phenomenon. Instead, the non-sociologist critic of the "professional project"[7] of bioethics can combine the perspectives in novel ways to reinforce the sense that the professionalization of ethics consultation services is an ominous development and a reversal of traditional democratic values.[8]

The sociological perspective on professionals and professional work most familiar in everyday discourse has been developed by Talcott Parsons.[9] This perspective develops a portrait of the "selfless" professional. In this view, the professional possesses expert theoretical knowledge that is acquired after a long period of adult socialization. This knowledge is then applied to solve client problems in some domain with a "high value salience" for members of the society. Here, the classic professions serve as an example of what "value salience" means concretely—medicine's domain is health; the law's, justice; and the clergy's, salvation. Without this application of expert knowledge, the client, who is described in this perspective as "incompetent," is unable to solve his or her problem.

Because, in this perspective, both professional and client share goals and values, no concern is paid to the manner in which the professional usurps the client's decision-making authority. First, since the client and professional both want the same thing—the client's return to health, the doing of justice on the client's behalf, or salvation of the client's soul—the professional is assumed to do naturally what the client wants. The assumption of value convergence makes paternalism a nonproblem. The professional's actions are simply an extension of the client's will. In this perspective, the client's seeking the professional's service is conflated with accepting the professional's plan. Second, the perspective assumes that the professional's authority to usurp client decision making is highly limited. Professional authority is not a highly generalized medium; rather, it is "functionally specific," limited to the domain of theoretical expertise. If, and when, professionals usurp lay authority, they do so only in a limited domain, as the client's agent, at the client's direction, and with the client's prior approval. A final safeguard against professionals overreaching the legitimate sphere of their authority is their socialization in a "service ethic." It is this expectation that the professional will act as the client's fiduciary that, when combined with a faith in the superiority of expert knowledge, allows this perspective on professionals to evade the questions of individual autonomy that are so central to bioethics.[10]

Another perspective on the nature of professional authority and work grew up alongside and in opposition to the highly idealized characterization described above. Developed by Everett C. Hughes and his students,[11] this perspective develops a portrait of the "selfish" professional. In this description, all the propositions about professionals and their work that make up the model of the "selfless" professional are inverted. So instead of granting any incontestable status to expert knowledge, this perspective questions claims to expert knowledge and separates claims of theoretical knowledge from applications of that knowledge. Professions, in this view, are an organization of similarly situated workers who convince the state to provide an exclusive "license" and "mandate" to provide services. As a result of this "license" and "mandate," professionals are able to control the production of services, and through this control create an artificial scarcity and reap monopolistic benefits. The long adult period of socialization and professional codes of ethics, said by those who view professional service romantically to guarantee virtuous service to others, is viewed quite skeptically by those who emphasize the self-interested dimensions of professional behavior.

> I wish to suggest that neither sociological analysis nor public policy is well served by defining ethicality as good intentions, expressed as a formal code or as attitudes. Rather, I wish to suggest that the most useful definition does not lie in codes or in attitudes. But in behavior at work. Just as I suggested that expertise assumes empirical status according to what the expert does in his work, so I now suggest that ethicality assumes empirical status of most consequence in the ways that the ethical occupation controls the performance of work. . . . *What professionals do represents their effective knowledge or expertise; how they regulate what they do in the public interest represents their effective service orientation or ethicality.*[12]

Few of the authors writing in this tradition find that the medical profession meets Freidson's test of ethicality. It is not merely that the social control of performance is lax and haphazard,[13] but also that the profession's justifications, explanations, and claims about its behavior frequently do not align with the behavior itself.

One example well illustrates the gap between the profession's claims to ethicality and its performance: namely, the ways in which information control is used to prevent patients' autonomy. This is a well-chosen example for the simplest of reasons. The empirical research reported here occurred before the institutionalization of current standards of informed consent, so this research indexes just how much of a difference bioethics has made and at the same time displays how toothless ethical codes can be in protecting patients' dignity. The earliest empirical work on the process of dying in hospitals indicated that great effort was exerted to make certain that patients did not know they were dying.[14] Physicians and, to be fair, the families of dying patients felt that such information would create untoward stress, would involve patients' "flooding out" emotionally,[15] and would, in general, make day-to-day patient management difficult.

What was true for the dying was true for other patients as well. Candor was in short supply. Physicians relied on patients' trust in the doctor's technical expertise and moral authority to guide treatment. The absence of information shared was a primary strategy of control. Fred Davis, for example, looked at how physicians manipulate uncertainty about time to recovery in order to manipulate patients. Davis sought "to distinguish between 'real' uncertainty as a clinical scientific phenomenon and the uses to which uncertainty—real or 'pretended,' 'functional' uncertainty—lends itself in the management of patients and their families by hospital physicians and other treatment personnel."[16]

Davis demonstrated that physicians and other treatment personnel feign uncertainty about the extent of and time to recovery long after such uncertainty has been resolved. This feigning of uncertainty, this dissembling, allows physicians to sustain an atmosphere of buoyant optimism, to motivate patients and their families to cooperate with arduous programs of physical therapy, and to prevent (or at least stall) patients and their families from dropping out of conventional therapy and taking up alternative therapies viewed as forms of unethical quackery by physicians who see their own evasions as ethical behavior in service of the patient's own good. Quint described the "information management practices" physicians and nurses used to avoid disclosing a breast cancer diagnosis to patients, and detailed how "both consciously and unconsciously the staff make use of strategies which limit patients' opportunity to negotiate for information."[17] Such strategies include the staff busying themselves with technical work, rotating frequently, and failing to become familiar with patients' prognoses.

In the Parsonsian perspective, professional expertise subserves the physician's fiduciary relationship with the patient. In the alternative perspective, professional expertise is viewed skeptically and ironically: physicians claim to deploy their skill, expertise, and power for the patient's benefit, but a close examination of behavior shows both claims and benefits to be dubious. For our purposes here, it is not so critical to decide which perspective is more valid.[18] Rather, our concern is to point out that the actions of certified licensed practitioners can be described in terms that celebrate the profession's contribution to the collective good or that question it in quite forceful turns. In one sense, the debate over the advisability of licensure and certification is the wrong debate in which to engage. What is more important to assess is a judgment that I shall leave for others: does ethics consultation contribute to the collective good, and if so, at what cost? The questions I am prepared to discuss here are why licensure and certification is inadvisable "at this time" and why I expect "at this time" to last for a very long time indeed.

Some Practical Difficulties with Licensure and Certification

In theory, occupational licensure and certification is a consumer protection measure. Presumptively, it serves to identify for consumers practitioners whose skills and competence have met some minimal tests and standards set by the community of practitioners. In theory again, licensure and certification is particularly necessary where knowledge and skills are esoteric, where lay judgment of services is either difficult or unreliable, and where the consequences of incompetence are grave. So, while both massage therapists and vascular surgeons may receive licenses and certificates, the process of licensure and certification has a social (as well as economic) meaning for surgeons that it does not have for masseurs. Both surgeons and masseurs may properly claim to be licensed and certified professionals. Both may take pride in those claims and in the efforts required to achieve that status. But, I would argue, those claims are more consequential for the surgeon than the masseuse. One way to think about licensure and certification for an ethics consultant is to ask: does ethical consultation more closely resemble massage or surgery? Of course, when ridiculous extremes frame rhetorical questions, there is not much drama in the answer. Below, in answering as I will, I do not mean to trivialize the work of ethical consultants or that of massage therapists, or to minimize the harm that can result from a bad consultation or an incompetent massage, or to deny the benefits of either when well-executed. Rather, I wish to discuss those dimensions of everyday practice that make it likely that licensure and certification for ethics consultants holds so little promise for the protection of the public welfare, the assurance of high-quality consultation, or the prevention of consultations of dubious value.

As a collectivity of consumers, we care, and care intensely, whether vascular surgeons are licensed and certified or not. Lay standards are not sufficiently fine-grained to distinguish competent technical performance. Lay standards may establish which vascular surgeons are louts or bores and which are kind and compassionate. But a highly skilled lout in this situation may do much good, while a charming incompetent may do much harm. Unfortunately, lay standards do not provide much guidance in assessing the technical skills of the surgeon. On the other hand, while professional massage therapists undoubtedly assess performance by different criteria than do lay users of their service, it is not clear how important those technical criteria are to lay users. Clients feel that either a massage helped or it did not. Licensing and certification in this case sends a signal to lay users about what kind of service to expect; but there is little to suggest that, within the class of licensed massage therapists—that is, the class of respectable and reputable suppliers of massage—lay evaluation is inadequate.

If we knew who the clients of ethics consultants were, if we knew what the goals of consultation were, arguments for or against licensing and certification would be easier to formulate, judgments easier to make. Still, there is no reason to think that lay standards would not be adequate to judge whether the service was competently provided or not. What, then, would licensing and certification provide in the case of ethics consultants? It would for certain limit the supply of servers, creating a presumptive monopoly for those with licenses and certificates. After all, if there were licensing and certification for ethics consultants, what institution would be willing to risk the legal liabilities incurred when personnel do not meet this minimal professional standard? But while privileging the credentials of some over others, would licensing and certification do anything to promise a higher-quality service?

The difficulties with making reasonable claims for licensure and certification center on the key points of contention for assessing the nature of professional work: namely, the nature of theory, its relation to practice, and the difficulty of establishing that the occupation in question serves the public good. Let us start with theory. One can make a reasonable claim that principlism—the flexible deployment and balancing of autonomy, beneficence, nonmaleficence, and justice—is the dominant paradigm in the field.[19] However, as many have noted, knowing the principles of principlism, mastering the theory, does not necessarily provide a reliable guide to action. Two problems present themselves. First, the values of principlism are but vague guides to action. As such, they are "essentially contestable"; articulating which values should guide action is one thing, demonstrating that this or that behavior truly embodies those values is another. That one can state the principles of principlism is not necessarily a guarantee that one knows either how to recognize which situations are problematic ethically or how to choose among those principles to produce ethics in action. In addition, while principlism is the dominant paradigm in bioethics, it is by no means the only one. Competing perspectives for resolving issues include (but are not limited to) casuistry, contractarian ethics, feminist ethics, narrative ethics, a phenomenological approach, and a variety of faith-based approaches. If we as a society were to license and certify ethics consultants, would we look for mastery of principlism or would we accept mastery of other paradigms as well? Or would we look for a more general mastery, what the ASBH report identifies as "core competencies" in the skill areas of ethical assessment, group process, and interpersonal relations, and then make certain that these existed along with a core knowledge of common bioethical issues and concepts?

Whichever way we chose to assess the theoretical knowledge of the ethics consultant, we would still face a second difficulty. We would have no assurance that this theoretical knowledge, however assessed, had any relation to outcomes, good, bad, or indifferent. In part, this is so because, despite a virtual consensus that ethics consultation is a good thing, there is a lack of clarity on both how consultation should be conducted and what consultation is intended to achieve. The position that ethics consultation is desirable is one with a fair amount of institutional support at this point. Since *Quinlan*, commentators have been nearly unanimous in their dislike for using judicial arenas for resolving conflicts of medical ethics. Courts rely on procedural rules not ethical arguments, are committed to adversarial process, have no specific competence in clinical matters, are burdened with overfull dockets without taking on questions of medical ethics, and have deliberative decision-making schedules that are not geared to the needs of the instant case. The suggestion of the *Quinlan* court (the New Jersey Supreme Court) that hospitals use ethics committees to resolve cases was given some teeth when the Joint Commission on Accreditation of Healthcare Organizations specified that organizations seeking its approval need to have in place a mechanism for resolving ethical conflicts. The JCAHO is silent on what form that mechanism needs to take and on what exactly is a conflict serious enough to require its use. Nonetheless, the JCAHO's standard has spurred the development of institutional ethics committees and furthered the role of ethics consultants.[20] Similarly, the American Hospital Association has strongly urged that its member organizations have in place a process for dealing with the "inevitable" ethical conflicts that arise in everyday contexts of care.

All of this urging from courts, commentators, accrediting bodies, and professional organizations is quite clear about what institutional ethics committees and ethics consultants are to do: namely, resolve conflict. What counts as an acceptable way for accomplishing this goal, however, remains unspecified. There are numerous modes for resolving conflict that presumptively would not pass any ethical muster, for example, the simple assertion of naked power: "We will do it this way because I say so." So, while the ultimate objective of ethics consultation may be to resolve conflict, how this objective is achieved is not unimportant. How, then, are we to judge the effectiveness of ethics consultation? What measures do we use? And, if we do not have something like a community-wide consensus about how to measure the effectiveness of ethics consultation (and presumably the consultants who assume some responsibility for them) and how to think about outcomes and process, then how can we license and certify committees or consultants? In this case, we would be granting the presumptive monopoly that licensing and certification provides absent any demonstration that any particular mode of thinking about ethical problems, any particular method of conducting consultations, yields better results than any other. Under those conditions, it is hard to understand the grounds for either granting or denying a license or certification to any applicant.

Some Philosophical Questions Raised by Licensure and Certification

But suppose the objections to licensing or certification stated so far either are horribly wrong-headed (there is an agreed-upon knowledge base for clinical ethics, a proper way to conduct an ethical consultation, and nothing mysterious about assessing the outcome of those consultations) or have been overcome. Let us suppose "this time" during which the task force found it inappropriate to consider licensing and certification has come to an end and we have arrived at some new time in which the arguments against licensing and certification have been overcome one by one. Further, let us assume the existence of some professional body with the standing, resources, and organizational capacity to administer the requisite tests for certifying or licensing ethics consultants. To strain the imagination just a tiny bit more, let us assume as well that we have a valid and reliable test of the theoretical knowledge and practical skills that an ethics consultant needs to possess.[21] Under those conditions, is licensing and certification a good idea? I obviously think not or I would not have bothered to frame such an elaborate set of requirements that, if met, would so clearly favor licensing and certification.

After all, if there is an occupational community of ethics consultants, what possible objection is there in its licensing and certifying its practitioners? What possible mischief is done in informing the lay public of who meets the standards of the professional community and who does not? As I search for an overall rationale to connect the various threats that I see in licensing and certification, I am aware of a sputtering inchoateness in my arguments, a quality of what about this, or that, or the next thing, that lends an air of unwavering unreasonableness to the presentation. For this, I apologize. Yet, I have had for some time a visceral dis-ease with the professionalization of bioethics.[22] I can place this dis-ease in a linguistic change.

When *bioethics* denoted a substantive domain, a set of common problems attended to by people who identified themselves as lawyers, philosophers, physicians, nurses, clergy, social workers, and social scientists and who viewed themselves as engaged in a common interdisciplinary enterprise, I felt no great discomfort with either the emergence of bioethics or its institutionalization in medical centers. But now that *bioethics* denotes those very same problems, but those engaged with them, whatever their disciplinary origin, identify themselves as bioethicists, the very developments that I applauded a few years earlier now seem more ominous. The identification of *bioethicist* as a disciplinary identity seems to me to signal the closing of the social and intellectual space that the substantive concerns of bioethics had promised to open up. In short, although it may be very much too late in the game for this sort of argument to have any persuasive force, licensing and certification of ethics consultants appears to me out of step with whatever leveling, democratic impulses originally motivated bioethics. The licensing and certification of clinical ethicists appears to me an antidemocratic move that narrows who can legitimately engage the questions of bioethics, what questions can be engaged, and what answers to those questions will be accepted as valid. As others have noted, each move in the professionalization of bioethics as an applied clinical specialty has the potential to supplant lay values with expert ones, as well as the potential to shrink the zone of individual autonomy. That this potential exists in the work of those who are among the most vociferous defenders of individual autonomy in society is ironic, to say the least. Nonetheless, as Freidson suggested in the passage quoted above with regard to assessing any occupation's ethics, actions and their consequences are weightier than intentions.

So, fiery rhetoric aside, what is the specific threat to the republic that licensing and certification of ethics consultants presents to democratic order? Since this is a slippery-slope sort of argument, we have to begin with an innocent slide that should allow enough rhetorical momentum for the alleged danger to become clear. Licensing and certification implies some sort of testing; that testing involves some selection from a likely list of routine suspects—a multiple-choice fund-of-knowledge component, an essay component, a practical simulated-conundrum component, and an "assessing the character of the character" interview. Preparation for this fateful ordeal will take place through degree programs that will begin to have a more rigid structure—what we need to know and teach becomes what counts for licensure and certification.[23] Licensing and certifying exams create a "de facto" closure to the field. Those domains not featured on the exam become, in the operation of things, less important than those that are so featured. The permeable disciplinary and substantive membrane separating that which is officially bioethics from all else becomes a much finer mesh. Approaches and topics that now find a home in bioethics face the possibility of being rejected as not what we need to know, not what the licensing and certifying bodies recognize as important. To the argument that the permeability of the membrane separating bioethics from other domains is becoming more fine-grained without licensing and certification, and that this is perhaps a natural consequence of the development of intellectual maturation, academic departments, and degree-granting programs, I would have no objection. However, I would add that licensing and certification would only accelerate an undesirable process and provide less incentive to support new approaches to old questions or to explore new questions within bioethics.

Beyond all this, within a domain that has explicitly trumpeted its commitment to leveling hierarchy—especially the asymmetric decision-making authority of doctor and patient—licensing and certification creates two new elite groups: first, within the group of those licensed and certified, there are the examiners and everyone else; second, there are those with licenses and certificates and those without. Given the requirements for qualifying to even take most licensing and certification examinations—so much course work of just this type, so many hours of just this sort of experience, so many testimonials from so many supervisors—this second elite stratifies in unintended as well as intended ways. Formal requirements are almost always legitimated rhetorically by reference to their favorable impact on standards and performance, with their resultant beneficial impact on the collective good. What advocates of formal requirements are less likely to mention is that such requirements restrict entry into a field by class, race, ethnicity, or gender. Nor are advocates forthcoming about how difficult the benefits of licensing and certification are to demonstrate.

But as baleful as are these consequences, as regrettable as is the dulling of the bioethical imagination, the loss of interdisciplinary vitality, or the formation of new elite groups, these are not the real challenge to democratic values posed by the licensing of ethics consultants. All are merely precursors, symptoms, or warning signs of the real threat posed by licensing and certification. This is a threat hard to state concisely—undoubtedly perceptive readers have by now noticed both this fact and my constant whining about it—but it is simply that the meaning of licensed and certified ethics consultants will be socially and organizationally overdetermined. That is to say, once we have licensed and certified ethics consultants, we will begin to feel that we must use them. The expert opinion will become required. As this happens, the lay voice, the values of the people, will come to be ignored. Even when the expert opinion is aligned with the lay choice, that lay choice will have no credibility or weight until ratified by the expert. And as, or if, this happens, one more domain critical to any schema of ordered liberty, one more domain that belongs in the control of ordinary, everyday people as they make life choices, ordinary and extraordinary, quotidian and unique, becomes the mystified domain of experts with specialized training, esoteric theories, fancy titles, and nicely appointed offices. When the process is complete, ordinary, everyday people lose their confidence and faith in their own ability to reason about their life choices, to know their preferences, and to make up their own minds. When the process is complete, ordinary, everyday citizens want the reassurance of an expert opinion. They become complicit in the usurpation of their own liberty. They become complicit because the presence of the licensed and certified ethics consultant has become "natural," the right thing to do. It is at this point that democratic values have become thoroughly eroded, that domination by professional expertise has become most complete. After all, those forms of social control that are most total, most pervasive, and most coercive are those that appear most "natural." It is when the need for, the legitimacy of, and the judgment by a licensed and certified ethics consultant feels most necessary that democratic values have been most eroded.[24]

In the end, licensing and certifying ethics consultants is a permanent solution to what should be seen as a temporary problem. If the need for ethics consultation is created by the need to educate doctors and patients about ways to talk with each other so that the everyday ethical problems that bedevil modern medicine can be resolved, then we can imagine a day when that education is complete, when new forms of dialogue, as well as new modes of decision making, have emerged. In this view, ethical consultants, and perhaps bioethicists, are merely transitional figures, guides as we move from old ways of conducting business in a presumably simpler time to new ways in an admittedly more complex world. But if, or when, we begin to license and certify ethics consultants, we discard this vision of bioethics as education and facilitation. We replace it with the ethics consultant as indispensable expert. This is something that, as I hope I have made clear, has the potential for much mischief.

A Temporizing Conclusion to Some Intemperate Arguments

Very early in the deliberations of the task force, we read some articles objecting to the existence and presence of ethics consultation. The arguments in these articles were forcefully stated and, in the mind of most task force members, quite extreme. During a break in our deliberations, one of the members sidled over to me and said something like, "You know if ethics consultation were done as these articles describe it, I would have the same objections. My problem is that I don't recognize ethics consulting as it is described in these articles." I imagine that many readers of this chapter have some of the same problems with my objections to licensing and certifying ethics consultants.

The ethics consulting that I have observed has been conducted by very, very decent people with the best of intentions. They work hard not to prejudge situations. They see their work as not so much making decisions as making sure that all relevant parties to a conflict have a voice and are heard. They try to make certain that all parties are aware of the full range of options. I have no doubt that, on many occasions, the mere knowledge that the disgruntled are able to seek an ethics consultation guarantees care more attentive to patients' rights than would be the case if ethics consultants were not available. I only have to think back to my fieldwork in the mid-1970s among surgeons,[25] and all those objectionable actions I observed that occurred with no public discussion, all those conflicts resolved with the simple assertion that "there are some decisions that only an attending surgeon can make," to see how much ethical consultation has changed the world for the better.

This being so, how can I object to the licensing and certification of ethical consultants, especially when the goal is merely to improve the quality of a needed service that appears to have made care more humane and promises to make it even more so in the future? Further, aware of how much good has been done by ethical consultants, how can I be so vehement—and, I must admit, that vehemence as it tumbled onto the page surprised me—and so dogmatic in my objections? In the final analysis, my objections to licensing and certification "at this time" and, to be fair, most probably at any future time, are the ones quoted at the beginning of this chapter, as stated so starkly at the conclusion of the ASBH report: the displacement of patients and providers as primary decision makers, the undermining of diversity within bioethics, the institutionalization of a particular morality, the difficulties in finding reasonable measures of competence that are then reasonably related to outcomes, and the administrative costs and consequences entailed in any schema for licensing and certification. To all those objections, I would add one more: it is hard for me to imagine that if licensing and certification were a step taken by the bioethics community that proved to be a mistaken step, we would have the capacity to recognize this mistake and correct it. Rather, I imagine us all constantly reminding ourselves that the theory and spirit of licensing and certification are quite correct, that we just need to work harder to get the practice of the thing right, that sometime soon we will get the bugs out, that we are merely at the beginning of what we all knew was going to be a difficult process. My worries, then, are less concerned with bioethics consultation, whatever its imperfections, as it is practiced now. Rather, my worries are about what ethics consultation might become under regimes of licensing and certification.

Notes

1. Society for Health and Human Values–Society for Bioethics Consultation: Task Force on Standards for Bioethics Consultation, *Core Competencies for Health Care Ethics Consultation: The Report of the American Society for Bioethics and Humanities* (Glenview, Ill.: American Society for Bioethics and Humanities, 1998), 31.
2. In general, there is a set of rather tendentious qualifications about the form ethics consulting takes, which I should mention here but will not. The most important of these is whether consulting is done by an individual or a committee. In general, unless stated otherwise, I assume that arguments about certification apply equally to individuals and committees. I do this fully recognizing that the licensing requirements and procedures for individuals and organizations are somewhat distinct.
3. ASBH report, 2.
4. J. Ross, "The Task Force Report: Comprehensible Forest or Unknown Beetles?" *Journal of Clinical Ethics* 10, no. 1 (1999):26.
5. C. L. Bosk, "Professional Ethicist Available: Logical, Secular, Friendly," *Daedalus* 128, no. 4 (1999): 47–68.
6. C. Rosenberg, "Meanings, Policies, and Medicine: On the Bioethical Enterprise and History," *Daedalus* 128, no. 4 (1999):44.
7. M.S. Larsen, *The Rise of Professionalism: A Sociological Perspective* (Berkeley: University of California Press, 1979).

8. G. Scofield, "The Least Dangerous Profession?" *Cambridge Quarterly of Healthcare Ethics* 2 (1993):417–48.

9. T. Parsons, *Essays in Sociological Theory* (New York: Free Press, 1949); T., Parsons, "Professions," in *International Encyclopedia of the Social Sciences* (New York: Macmillan, 1968).

10. D. Crane, *The Sanctity of Social Life: Physicians' Treatment of Critically Ill Patients* (New York: Russell Sage Foundation, 1975).

11. E. C. Hughes, *The Sociological Eye, Book Two: Selected Papers on Work, Self, and the Study of Society* (Chicago: Aldine-Atherton, 1971); H. Becker, "The Nature of a Profession," in *Educating for the Professions* (Chicago: National Society for the Study of Education, 1962), 27–46; E. Freidson, *The Profession of Medicine: A Study in the Sociology of Applied Knowledge* (1970; Chicago: University of Chicago Press, 1988); E. Freidson, *Doctoring Together* (New York: Elsevier, 1975); E. Goffman, *Asylums* (New York: Doubleday, 1961).

12. E. Freidson, *Profession of Medicine,* 1988 ed., 360–61, emphasis in the original.

13. E. Freidson and B. Rhea, "Processes of Control in a Company of Equals," in *Medical Men and Their Work,* ed. E. Freidson and J. Lorber (Hawthorne, N.Y.: Walter de Gruyter, 1971); Freidson, *Doctoring Together.*

14. B. Glaser and A. Strauss, *Awareness of Dying* (Chicago: Aldine, 1965); B. Glaser and A. Strauss, *Time for Dying* (Chicago: Aldine, 1968); B. Glaser and A. Strauss, *Status Passages* (Chicago: Aldine-Atherton, 1971).

15. E. Goffman, *The Presentation of Self in Everyday Life* (Garden City, N.J.: Anchor-Doubleday, 1959).

16. F. Davis, "Uncertainty in Medical Diagnosis: Clinical and Functional," *American Journal of Sociology* 66 (1960):259–67.

17. J. Quint, in Freidson and Lorber, *Medical Men and Their Work,* 232; J. Quint, "Institutionalized Practices of Information Control," *Psychiatry: Journal for the Study of Interpersonal Processes* 28, no. 2 (1965):119–32.

18. A. Abbott, *The System of the Professions: An Essay on the Division of Expert Labor* (Chicago: University of Chicago Press, 1988). There is a third perspective on professions: namely, Abbott's "system" of professions (ibid.). This focuses on the competition among professional occupations for dominance (e.g., the struggle among psychologists, pastoral counselors, social workers, and psychiatrists for professional "jurisdiction" over mental health services). Since our concern here is less with competition between and among groups to provide a service and more with the nature of the qualifications of any individual from any occupational background, Abbott's framework is not immediately useful. However, should licensing and certification come to pass at some later date, Abbott's framework would be a useful tool for helping us understand not only why this occurred but also why whatever requirements were adopted took the shape that they did.

19. T. L. Beauchamp and J. Childress, *Principles of Biomedical Ethics* (New York: Oxford University Press, 1979); T. Chambers, *The Fiction of Bioethics: Cases as Literary Texts* (New York: Routledge, 1999); P. Wolpe, "The Triumph of Autonomy in American Bioethics," in *Bioethics and Society: Constructing the Ethical Enterprise,* ed. R. Devries and J. Subedi (Upper Saddle River, N.J.:

Prentice Hall, 1998); B. Hoffmaster, "Can Ethnography Save the Life of Medical Ethics?" *Social Science and Medicine* 35 (1992):1421–31.

20. C. L. Bosk and J. Frader, "Institutional Ethics Committees: Sociological Oxymoron, Empirical Black Box," in Devries and Subedi, *Bioethics and Society.*

21. The easiest objection to the hypothetical conditions I have just set for ethics consultants is that the bar has been set too high. In fact, I am making the licensing and certification of ethics consultants rest on conditions that other occupations with licensing and certification are not required to fulfill. In essence, the objection is that I have made the perfect the enemy of the good. This is indeed possible, but since I believe licensing and certification has the potential for achieving more mischief than good, I am more than willing to set very stringent criteria. I recognize that those with a sunnier view of licensing and certification are probably willing to provide less stringent criteria.

22. C. L. Bosk, *All God's Mistakes: Genetic Counseling in a Pediatric Hospital* (Chicago: University of Chicago Press, 1992), esp. chap. 6.

23. Here it is important to remember that however cynical those "grandfathered" out of the initial licensing and certification ordeal may be about how well that ordeal measures whatever we take to be core competence, the test itself will be fateful for those who have to take it: it will influence their employment opportunities, their life-chances, in real ways. If licensing and certification exams for ethical consultants take hold, and if the results of that taking hold follow the patterns of other institutionalized exam passage points in our society, we will have created three new growth industries: (1) the exam makers, graders, and administrators; (2) the exam-preparation services; and (3) the cultural critics of the whole process. As I suspect this chapter has made more than abundantly clear, I am angling for a position on the ground floor of that third line of enterprise.

24. After all this overheated prose, I think an even-minded critic might object as follows: doesn't this all depend on what the expert would recommend? That I think not is obvious. My reasons may not be so clear. Simply stated, organizing care so that ethical values and individual autonomy rely on the wisdom exercised by a professional expert embedded in a bureaucratic organization not only feels risky; it removes power and authority from the patient in order to preserve the patient's power and authority. The entire process seems to me to be filled with internal contradictions—individual autonomy is difficult to regulate bureaucratically.

25. C. L. Bosk, *Forgive and Remember: Managing Medical Failure* (Chicago: University of Chicago Press, 1979).

THREE

Institutional Ethics Committees

SOCIOLOGICAL OXYMORON, EMPIRICAL BLACK BOX

Charles L. Bosk and Joel Frader

Despite the collective belief that medical practice rests on solid scientific grounds, change in medicine typically comes about in a haphazard, complex fashion. New practices often constitute reactions to external social, political, and economic forces, rather than adoption of technical advances. Certainly, the major restructuring of health-care practices begun in the late 1980s and early 1990s—*integrated networks* brought about through mergers and acquisitions with promised efficiencies of scale; *managed care,* with its purported elimination of wasteful, inefficient, and unnecessary care; cost savings through health maintenance organizations, which supposedly flow from prevention rather than more expensive rescue—all provide examples of changes based on theory rather than systematically established grounds. Other wholesale changes in practice follow changes in fashion among leaders in health care professions prior to concrete demonstration of benefit. Examples in medicine include the introduction of coronary care units (Bloom and Peterson 1973), the use of fetal monitoring (Hess 1980; Nelson et al. 1996), and radical surgical treatment for breast cancer (Fisher et al. 1985).

Chapter 3 was originally published as Charles L. Bosk and Joel Frader, "Institutional Ethics Committees: Sociological Oxymoron, Empirical Black Box," in *Bioethics and Society: Constructing the Ethical Enterprise,* ed. Raymond DeVries and Janardan Subedi. (Upper Saddle River, N.J.: Prentice Hall, 1998), 94–116.

This process—transformations in practice absent persuasive evidence of efficacy—is now being repeated with the institutionalization of what Renée Fox (1989) has called the "bioethics movement." We refer here to the establishment of small groups in hospitals, nursing homes, and the like, known as hospital or institutional ethics committees (IECs), to respond to moral issues and to clinical ethics consultation (CEC) services. The fact that IECs and CEC are the mechanisms to resolve multiple tensions and conundrums in delivering modern care is in itself not surprising, as each adopts well-worn structural responses to problems of social control. In most health care settings, CEC uses familiar methods modeled on medical practice (La Puma and Schiedermayer 1991) to deal with patient, family, or staff behavior that deviates from the expected or from what authorities prefer. In many ways, IECs simply extend long-established patterns of peer and community oversight and provide a mechanism for educating those in the institution and for generating institutional policy (Ross 1986). In other ways, IECs and CEC are a novel response to the exquisitely difficult, painful existential dilemmas of contemporary medical care.

Institutional Ethics Committees: Historical Background and Context

Since the late 1960s, responding to the memory of Nazi medical experiments and the more recent scandalous behavior of researchers in the United States, the federal government has required institutions that receive federal research support to have in place an institutional review board (IRB). These committees, according to federal regulations, must include at least seven members, including a scientist, a practicing physician, a nurse, and one community "representative." The IRB's stated role is to ensure that proposed experimentation falls safely within both professional and community norms for acceptable conduct. Operationally, this often means a limited review in practice. IRBs focus on the risk-benefit ratio of proposed research and the extent to which consent forms are both understandable and complete. IRB review is completely forward looking and relies on an honor system; there is rarely, if ever, surveillance to assess compliance. Nonetheless, since their introduction, IRBs have provided review of research protocols. In doing so, these committees expanded the circle of those who can legitimately participate in the collective oversight of biomedical and behavioral research.[1]

In this light the emergence of IECs seems little more than an extension of an organizational innovation into a new domain. But, of course, matters are

more complicated than they appear. Thinking of IECs as a linear development of earlier forms of professional oversight and control misses much of
what is new in this organizational form and certainly misses the important
ways that IECs differ from IRBs. Most significantly, it discounts the fact that
IRBs were largely the product of federal mandates, which regulated their
membership, their functions, and, even to a degree, their procedures. IECs,
as we will soon see, grew in a much more free-form way, with no requirements for representation, no clear delimited tasks, no set procedures, and
no formal mandate for coming into being (Cransford and Doudera 1984).
Institutions were compelled to have IRBs if they wished to retain federal
support; there was no similar incentive to encourage recalcitrant institutions into developing IECs. The recent requirement of the Joint Commission
on the Accreditation of Health Care Organizations that institutions seeking
accreditation have a mechanism for resolving problems in clinical ethics is
silent on what that process should be. If IECs are the proper mechanism,
how they should then be structured and function or, more to the heart of
the matter, what standards or processes the IEC should adopt for reaching
substantive closure on moral matters is unspecified.

Origins are difficult to trace with precision. How beginnings are located,
what counts as an institutional antecedent to IECs, and what forerunners
are ignored tell us more about the intent of the analyst than it informs us
about IECs. If the analyst tells the story in such a way that IECs are seen as
an extension of earlier organizational forms, then one can expect a Whig history of medical ethics. Each moment is a monument in the march of progress
that allows greater weight to be put on ethical values at the bedside. On the
other hand, if the account emphasizes the work necessary to impose these
strange and new forms of oversight into alien and uninviting territory, then
one will hear a tale in which bioethicists and those concerned with a more
broad, holistic view of medical action are courageous reformers, expanding
human liberties in domains hostile and resistant to such expansion. There is
a substantial validity to both accounts, making it a difficult narrative problem to tell both at the same time.

This explanatory difficulty aside, to explain and analyze the rise of IECs,
it is necessary to begin somewhere. Three early developments are worthy
of mention.[2] As Renée Fox and Judith Swazey (1974) reported, citizens'
committees in Seattle formed to allocate scarce kidneys among the multiple potential recipients faced many ethical dilemmas and can be seen as
a forerunner of current committees. However, it is worth noting that such
committees faced enormous pressures trying to reach consensus, never ar-

ticulated standards for decision making, and eventually disbanded, an out-come perhaps helped along by considerable adverse publicity. An important feature of all these groups was the sharp focus on case-by-case decisions. The committees functioned, in effect, as clinical consultants. As with most such clinical activity, neither the social rules that structured the consultation nor the philosophical and social values assumptions that shaped the decisions were explicit.

Next, there were the controversies surrounding nontreatment in neonatal intensive care, stimulated by the report of Raymond Duff and A. G. M. Camp-bell (1973) at Yale–New Haven Hospital. These authors revealed their private troubles and decision making as a way to force a public reevaluation of the operating procedures and underlying presuppositions that tended to support more, or excessive, treatment rather than permit the deaths of patients with poor prognoses. At Yale then, there were no ethics committees, but there was merely public recognition of the need for them. At about that time, others had begun to suggest that ethically focused intrainstitutional groups might begin to confront the growing disjunction between capacity and rationale for life-extending treatment. The publication in 1971 of *The Medico-Moral Guide* of the Catholic Bishops (of Canada) recommended the formation of medico-moral committees in Catholic health care facilities. Although the guide iden-tified the absence of sufficient personnel trained in theology and ethics and the lack of involvement of hospital personnel as potential problems, hoped for benefits from committee formation included education of staff and the widening of the moral dialogue about the proper mission of modern health care institutions. In 1976 a lawyer and a pediatrician (Robertson and Fost 1976) suggested committees might help address some of the ethical and le-gal questions that treatment-limitation practices raised. There was, then, a call from several quarters to pay special attention to ethical problems in the domain of health care, especially in regard to the increasing frequency of di-lemmas consequent to advancing medical technology.

Arguably, the single biggest impetus to the formation of ethics commit-tees came in 1976 when the Supreme Court of New Jersey, in the Quinlan case, adopted a proposal in the literature by Karen Teel (1975). The court suggested that hospitals form ethics committees to keep disputes, such as the one before them, out of the courts. Three features of this landmark deci-sion are worth noting:

1.   The New Jersey court was silent about how these committees should be organized and how their deliberations would prevent litigation.

2. The court distorted Teel's recommendation and, in so doing, created some confusion about whether the committees were to concern themselves with medical matters, such as prognosis and futility, or with morals.

3. It is unclear how committee arbitration squares with the right, articulated by the Quinlan court, of individuals or their surrogates to make private medical decisions. Nonetheless, here was a court in a widely publicized case calling for a major change in how ethical dilemmas were managed.

The judicial call for peer review lifted the question of limiting life-sustaining treatment from the exclusive purview of the physician-patient relationship but left unclear the justification and best method(s) for such interventions. Similar conceptual and procedural confusion prevailed during and after 1982–85, a period of somewhat frenetic federal regulatory initiatives and congressional action invoking infant-care review committees to oversee treatment in cases of "handicapped" newborns. These developments followed in the wake of the Baby Doe case from Bloomington, Indiana. More recent legislation (in Maryland) and proposed regulation (New York state) requiring ethics committees to have some sort of consultative role in morally problematic cases have not settled a host of legal and philosophical questions of where IECs (should) fit in. As instruments of social control, the effectiveness of ethics committees seems to have been somewhat constrained by questions about the lawful and moral grounds for groups of strangers to intervene in medical decisions typically negotiated among patients, their loved ones, their surrogates, and treating professionals (Lo 1987; Fleetwood et al. 1989).

Ethics Consultation: Historical Background

The foregoing actually tracks much of the development of CEC, in that a large fraction of the consultative practice in medical ethics first occurred, at least in any formalized sense, through and by ethics committees. There is no easy separation of the origins of either. But there was another avenue of approach leading to CEC: the incorporation of theologians, philosophers, and occasionally others from the humanities (including sociologists) into clinical teaching programs in medical schools and some residency (especially family practice) programs, in the 1960s and 1970s (Fletcher et al. 1989; Rothenberg 1989). To the extent that these "moral experts" became confidants and advice givers to clinicians grappling with real cases, rather than individuals who used the material presented on rounds to illustrate the general value and validity of ethical analysis, CEC was emerging in situ.

The appearance of nonclinicians, who some clinicians came to rely on, seems to have touched one or more sensitive nerves, leading to a contentious debate about what sorts of individuals might legitimately claim the mantle of consultant (Zaner 1993). We need not rehash that debate, but we should note that the question of how much clinical knowledge and skill CEC requires remains unsettled. Of course, how much and what sorts of knowledge and skill such a consultant ought to have (for example, philosophical, theological, mediation, legal, interactional, and small-group behavior) is an equally unresolved question, though these areas seem not to have created as much heat. That having been said, at least one prominent critic (Scofield 1993) claims that the very idea of *anyone* aspiring to the title of ethics consultant so offends our (political) tradition of individual liberty in a pluralistic society that we should quash any attempt to legitimize the role. These important questions—of what collection of characteristics constitute, and whether or how our society might endorse, the establishment of a new, historically complex profession (in the sense of having decidedly heterogeneous origins)—stand before us in the late 1990s. Indeed, one of us (CLB) sits on a blue-ribbon panel under the sponsorship of the Society for Health and Human Values and the Society for Bioethics Consultation, which is funded by the Greenwall Foundation, to deliberate on this very set of questions.[3]

Problematic Social Features of Ethics Consultation

BY COMMITTEE

In their way, ethics committees are an illustration of a sociological principle of Simmel—that of negative solidarity. It is relatively easy for groups to come together to identify what is wrong—in this case, inadequate attention paid to the ethical dimension of clinical care. Agreement often dissolves, however, when members of the group begin to pose remedies. Because our focus here is on the matter of the clinical consultative role of IECs, we will note some of the problems of committees relative to the consultative function. Among the issues are the following: the membership of the IEC, the kind of authority consultative activities ought to be regarded as having, and the procedures for organizing consultative activities.

Membership · Each institution has its own procedures for establishing membership on ethics committees. In some, the committees are open to volunteers. While this may ensure a certain level of motivation, we might wonder about how self-selection operates here. Who volunteers to be an ethical watchdog in an institution, and why? Of course, other means of selection are just as suspect. Appointment by administration raises questions of independence and of whose interest the committee serves. Election—given the gravity of the tasks—appears unseemly. Further, no method of selection does much to ensure that committee members possess the requisite expertise and knowledge base.[4]

The hospital is a complex formal organization; it is not clear who in the ranks should serve on ethics committees. Presumably, the more inclusive a committee, the better its chances of expressing a consensus, assuming we accept, as Jonathan Moreno (1995) argues, the importance of consensual agreement. But, there are many ways to be inclusive. Some ethics committees have top administrators and even members of the board of trustees. Their presence may send a message about the importance of ethics in or to the institution, but surely their participation can also inhibit the free flow of ideas. Many ethics committees include hospital legal counsel. To the extent that such attorneys can help clarify the inevitable questions of law that arise in ethically troublesome cases, hospital counsel can help the process work more efficiently. However, because the fiduciary responsibility of the hospital's legal staff is to advocate for positions protecting the hospital's interests, as opposed to the interests of individual employees or professional staff or the interests of patients and their loved ones, potential exists for (unacknowledged) conflict of interest to mar moral discourse. In addition, the well-known tendency of legal opinions to quiet if not quash discussion, given physicians' pervasive fear of litigation, may also undermine ideal moral problem solving.

How many physicians and how many nurses does a committee need? Which classes of workers do we include, and in what proportions? Do we seek out clinically essential people from the shop floor, such as respiratory therapists who deal with many of the patients whose right-to-die questions vex modern medicine? What of patient representation? Is it necessary or somehow beside the point? Is community participation as (symbolically) necessary here as it is with IRBs, or do the different missions of the two bodies signal different needs with regard to input by nonhospital personnel? This multitude of questions is not an idle listing of potential problems. Membership indicates who can speak and whose opinions are counted or discounted. Membership may determine even which issues are seen as legitimate ethical concerns and which are not. After all, both Renée Anspach (1993) and Daniel Chambliss (1996) have argued that a great many issues interpreted as ethical problems are merely structural disagreements among workers unequal in power, in different ranks, with different core tasks, and with disparate role-bound moralities. In this view, the label *ethical* legitimates a disagreement that the organizational actor with greater rank and authority could otherwise dismiss. To sharpen this point, we note that ethical problems within hospitalized care have arisen coincident in time with greater militancy among nurses to have their professional authority and expertise acknowledged. So, saying that a hospital has an ethics committee tells us very little unless we know as well who serves on the committee and under what authority.

Authority for and of consultation · It is worth recalling that part of the rationale of the Quinlan court's advocacy for ethics committees was to create an alternative arena, besides the courts, for resolving these dilemmas. To the extent that IECs are seen as carrying the authority of quasi-legal bodies, substituting for more formal (and expensive) procedures in the judicial system, one needs to worry about two probable consequences. First, as noted previously, invocations of "the law" in medical contexts tend to preempt more wide-ranging considerations, specifically those of moral import, which of course leads to missing the point of almost any kind of CEC. Thus, having an underlying legal motive for consultation both gives the process more clout than it might otherwise have and undermines the substantive ethics discourse. Second, as some have noted (Lo 1987; Fleetwood and Unger 1994), committee processes in hospitals typically do not entail the procedural safeguards—*due process* to use the legal system's term—that formal court proceedings typically include (see below).

But again, the social ramifications of authorizing IEC intervention are complex. The IEC can become, intentionally or otherwise, a mechanism for "cooling the mark out," just as an IRB can be (Levine 1983). Patients and their families now have another layer between them and a public complaint should they and their caregivers have a disagreement about what constitutes appropriate treatment. Thus, IECs may keep cases out of court, but this is not necessarily the same as having autonomy respected, ethical action ensured, or justice done. IECs may actually make it easier for physicians to override the wishes of patients and their families. A division of labor occurs: hospital physicians can focus on technical matters and take care of the patient's physiological demands; everything else can be "reduced" to ethics by physicians uncomfortable or ill equipped to deal with interpersonal or moral subtleties and then turfed to a specialized committee.[5] A couple of examples have been published by one group. Each case involved a child who physicians felt had received "enough" treatment. In the first instance, physicians concluded that it would not be appropriate to again use intensive care for a profoundly mentally disabled child with seizures and recurrent pneumonia (Paris et al. 1990). The child's mother disagreed and requested mechanical ventilation and other therapy that would sustain the child's life. The physicians took the case to the IEC, which supported and agreed to back them and the institution in a court action. In the second instance, a child had developed severe acute respiratory failure and did not respond to conventional therapy (Paris et al. 1993). The physicians agreed to a trial of extracorporeal membrane oxygenation (ECMO) as a last-ditch effort to permit recovery. However, as they embarked on the use of ECMO, they told the family that the treatment would be time limited. As the allotted time expired, not only without lung recovery but with other organ system failure developing as well, the family requested that ECMO be continued. Again, the physicians took the case to the IEC, claiming they had no obligation to provide "futile" treatment. The IEC again supported the physicians. If one can get beyond what is the "right" thing to do in these cases, it is not difficult to see how one could view them as instances where a powerful group of (mostly) professionals, the IEC, simply chose to support one value system (invested in efficient use of medical resources and a particular view of the quality of life) over another (invested in the value of biological human life itself and the particular lives of the unfortunate children, regardless of their mental state) held by those with much less institutional and social power, families of patients.

Procedures for organizing consultations · As we have already noted, keeping ethics cases in an IEC and out of the court also means giving up the legal system's elaborate protections for aggrieved parties. Committees are not bound to use specific rationales to arrive at decisions, need not observe any particular rules of evidence, nor need to announce or justify their decisions in any detail. Of course, we have no empirical evidence that such a lack of rules matters, and there are, naturally, advantages to hospital-based, rather than judicial, procedures. An IEC (or individual consultant) may have the ability to be sensitive to situational nuance, to act swiftly, and to bring to bear clinical experience that judges lack; committees can be informal, nonintimidating, and flexible. These qualities, if realized, do seem to suggest IECs can be a good substitute for moving into the courts.

But, as long as IECs operate behind closed doors, as Bernard Lo (1987) has pointed out, there is no way to tell whether they provide concrete advantages over more accountable processes, like those in the court system. In a very peculiar way, IECs reverse a trend in contemporary U.S. society toward more open systems with greater equality at the very same time that they seem to instantiate them. The very absence of any procedural standards makes it very difficult for outsiders to know how to evaluate the claim that the decision reached in a given case was endorsed by the IEC.

Individual ethics committees may or may not be clear on any of the following issues: who has the right to initiate a CEC; who has the right to appear before an ethics committee engaged in a consultation; how the group arrives at its decisions; how decisions are communicated (orally, in writing, in the medical record) and to whom (professionals only, patients and families as well as professionals). Not only are the internal workings of the ethics committee vexed, there are similarly tangled issues of the committee's relation to the hospital and larger environment.

Other issues include but are not limited to the confidentiality of deliberation—are committee findings and recommendations discoverable in malpractice actions? In addition, one can ask how proactive versus how reactive should committees be. That is, should all cases of a certain type receive prospective oversight or retrospective oversight, or should the IEC become involved in a case only when asked to comment on a specific concern. The Baby Doe law and regulations raise this issue fairly starkly. Should every neonatal case in which physicians and/or families considered forgoing treatment be brought to an infant care review committee? Perhaps IEC investigation should occur only with those cases typically thought of in terms of "handicapping conditions," such as those involving chromosomal abnormalities like Down syndrome (trisomy 21), or recognized clinical associations (syndromes) without a clear genetic basis. In fact, states (the only parties directly affected by the federal law) and hospitals have responded in a wide variety of ways. In some places, IEC involvement is mandated in various types of cases; elsewhere, the IEC only becomes involved if asked by a party in a particular case. In some places, case review is inclusive but only occurs retrospectively—that is, after clinical judgments have been arrived at and a disposition made.

Different modes of committee organization reflect different organizational understandings of what ethics committees are supposed to do and on whose behalf they are supposed to do it. If access to case consultation by a committee is limited only to physicians, or does not allow patient or family testimony, and conveys its opinions through letters to physicians that do not become part of the medical record, this reflects a very different understanding of organizational mission than a process whereby anyone can refer a case, in which all are allowed to give testimony and all recommendations appear as a note in the hospital chart. Herein lies a major problem. If ethics committees increase legal liability by revealing disputes about the proper standard of care, then we might expect that use of them would be at best reluctant On the other hand, when heeding the recommendations of committees is optional, members may well ask what the point of committee involvement might be. The proper balance between consent and coercion has yet to be found. It is one thing to put ethics committees in place; it is clearly quite another to ensure that they are taken seriously.

BY INDIVIDUAL CONSULTANT

The general concerns about consultation by committee also apply to consultations by individuals (or small teams of committee members). We can consider qualifications rather than membership, as well as matters of authority for consultation and the procedures to be followed.

Qualifications · As previously stated, precisely who qualifies as a consultant has by no means been settled. The necessary background, in terms of formal education or mastery of a body of knowledge and set of skills, remains controversial. Looking beyond formal characteristics of the consultant, of course, we should not ignore social status. There are in this area, as with other aspects of the actual doing of clinical ethics, few data to help us understand, for example, whether physician-ethicists versus nurse-ethicists versus philosopher-ethicists versus lawyer-ethicists (and so on) are especially "successful" (never mind how one might try to determine that) in helping resolve ethics disputes or in educating the public or institutional staff members about major issues in health care ethics. One can reasonably infer from the literature on consultation (as we do from our own experience, see Frader 1992) that physicians prefer to deal with physician-ethicists and nurses favor nurse-ethicists or specially organized nursing ethics committees. What this means—that is, whether it represents more than occupational solidarity or simply suggests that occupationally similar consultants communicate best with those with matching backgrounds—remains unclear. Skepticism about the inherent superiority (however defined) of one sort of consultant over another seems in order.

Authority · Regarding the authority of consultants to do their work, the issues may be somewhat more sharply focused than with a committee. After all, one of the advantages of having a committee is the opportunity to diffuse responsibility across statuses, across occupations, and sometimes across employers (that is, some on the IEC work for themselves, others for the hospital, others for a university, others may not be employed at all). If all the ethical weight of a situation falls on a single individual, how much more need we be concerned about whether that person reports directly to an administrator, an ethics committee, or some sort of clinical authority? Does it matter if the consultant is compensated by the hospital or through his or her faculty position at the affiliated university? Does it matter if the consultative activity results in a charge to the patient? These questions raise an additional level of concern, beyond the institutional bylaws or state legislation or regulations that support consultative activity, about agency. If the consultant is salaried by the hospital or the hospital pays for his or her "piecework," it seems legitimate to ask about the consultants' loyalties, as we would ask about the participation of hospital legal counsel on the ethics committee. There is an assumption in much of the CEC literature that consultants are "patient advocates," a mantle claimed by just about everyone these days, but the basis for that role seems both ideologically and structurally unclear in most instances.

Procedures · Rather than asking various parties to appear before a committee in a hearing-like setting, typically individual consultants or small teams go to the clinical setting to meet with interested parties. Assuming this is possible in a place ensuring reasonable privacy, it may offer a sociological and political advantage of, at least, appearing to accommodate to the needs of those directly involved. But there is, of course, a prior set of questions. Who will the consultant seek out, and how will the consultant approach such individuals? If the person or persons requesting consultation has qualms about the reaction of others, especially the attending physician, the requestor(s) may not want to discuss the consultation directly and openly. Most institutions require that the attending physician be notified of a CEC involving her or his patient, and some institutions still require attending physician approval/acceptance of the consultation. But that doesn't settle the question of *who* should notify attendings and whether the identity of the requestor must be disclosed.

These tensions also involve other aspects of consultative process. If, as is often the case, it appears that disputes can be managed by better communication among the involved parties and that a meeting or meetings of such individuals could be helpful, the consultant has to help overcome fears and other resistance to getting people together and then manage or mediate the discussion session. No matter what else, such procedures differ substantially from the quasi-judicial process often invoked in consultation by IECs, clearly call for different skills by those charged to lead in the matter, and have different sorts of implications for institutional social interaction during and after a consultation.

Sociological Interest in Ethics Consultation

Two features of CEC are immediately interesting.[6] First is the relative neglect of this development by sociologists. For some time now, sociologists have written critically of how health care professionals have used their expertise to narrow patient's options, disattend patient or family preferences, and in general overwhelm the will of sick persons and their loved ones. Unfortunately, the medical practice that we essentialize in this manner may not accurately reflect the current world of hospital practice. Little attention has been paid to whether changes in recent years—like the use of ethics committees and consulting ethicists and new legal rules (for example, the Patient Self-Determination Act, PSDA), which in theory provide a more muscular version of informed consent regarding such things as do-not-resuscitate orders—alter the traditional conception of the dominant professional and the compliant patient.[7]

There has been a remarkable increase in what might be termed the *epidemiology of ethics*—health services–type research conducted about the impact, if any, of advance medical directives, in accord with the PSDA or hospital policy, and whether the preferences of elderly or dying patients for end-of-life care are known or used by health care professionals or potential surrogates (Uhlmann et al. 1988; Zweibel and Cassel 1989; McCrary and Botkin 1989; Tomlinson et al. 1990; Danis et al. 1991; Sehgal et al. 1992; Stelter et al. 1992; Hare et al. 1992). There have also been surveys of "users" of CEC that address satisfaction with the process (La Puma 1987; La Puma et al. 1988; Perkins and Saathoff 1988; La Puma et al. 1992; McClung et al. 1996). Regrettably, none of this research ought properly be called sociological. The empirical studies typically have been done by insiders who are often some of the same individuals who lobbied for or against the policy changes and/or implemented them. The sociological studies that have looked at how ethics enter the world of the hospital bedside all precede the institutionalization of the ethics function in roles or committees (for examples, see

Zussman 1992, Anspach 1993, Fox and Swazey 1992, Bosk 1992; for a general discussion of these works and the relation of ethnographies of medical practice and bioethics, see Chambliss 1996, Frank 1995, Crigger 1995, or DeVries 1995).[8]

The absence of research here is particularly noteworthy in light of the joint commission regulations that, as we have noted, spurred the development of IECs. The fact that those regulations require only that hospitals have in place a "process" for dispute resolution surely created a situation where the variety of responses might shed some interesting light on the relationship between institutional structure and mission and the way institutions "handle" ethics. This lack of empirical attention is all the more surprising given the penchant of sociology to investigate the unintended consequences of planned social change and the divergence of organizational blueprints from everyday operations.

In addition, the process by which a new professional segment achieves legitimacy, successfully claims turf, and defines its domain of competence is of continuing interest to students of the professions.[9] Alternatively, the competition between scientific-technological rationales for action and humanistic models informed by philosophic or religious systems is fundamental to sociologists of culture, as is the construction of ethical authority. After all, there is little gainsaying that as a formal organizational actor in the modern hospital, the professional ethicist, whether in the guise of ethics committee or individual consultant, is a rather recently created role, the very existence of which challenges some of the clinical power and authority assumed by the attending physician in the context of the physician-patient relationship.

At the same time, the sociological literature suggests that the ethical authority these new actors claim to have is a poor substitute for the authority of science. Historically, moral authority is a type presumptively in retreat in a technologically complex, bureaucratic, and secular world. Why is it reappearing now, especially in that most modern of postmodern organizations—the tertiary care medical center? There is an empirical puzzle here that embarrasses our theories. So what is going on? How did this new (yet very old-fashioned looking) form of power and authority arise? Who are these "beeper" ethicists at the bedside, and why do others seek their advice? At the very least, the rationales by which authority is claimed, the domains in which these claims are accepted, and those in which it is resisted deserve our attention.

No better topic would seem to exist for looking at these issues than the institutionalization of ethical consultation. Here individual experts or committees either invade or are invited into the private space of the physician-patient relationship to discuss what course of action best satisfies the demands of morality as well as the question of how well—if at all—the demands of morality, professional customs and standards, and legal requirements can be harmonized. Phrasing the issue this way, of course, poses a problem. In writing of ethical consultation in problematic circumstances, or of bioethics more generally, there is a tendency to write as if all ethical problems are the result of conflict between physician and patient over what is the proper course of action. It is a convenient shorthand to write this way. The empirical world is of course more complex. Some conflicts and their attendant requests for consultation are intraprofessional—different specialty groups of physicians disagree among themselves about what proper action is; some are intrafamilial—brothers and sisters, children and parents argue over the bedside about who knows best what the patient, now unable to articulate a preference, really wanted; some are inter-professional—professional actors (for example, doctors and nurses) each with their own definition of professional mission disagree. Ethical disputes in the hospital do not even require two parties locked in a disagreement. A single individual, uncertain about the course of action, may clearly see the branches of the decision tree, feel lost in the ethical forest, and then request a consultation. Here there is a meeting for resolving conflict, but the conflict is intrapsychic. Finally it is worth noting that more than a few ethical troubles are created because the three spheres of morality, professional custom, and law are in conflict with one another.

So, whether for its theoretic or empirical attractions, one would think sociologists would be tripping all over themselves either explaining how ethical authority is socially constructed or superintending its deconstruction. One would think, to borrow David Rothman's evocative phrase, that we would insert ourselves and our analytic capabilities among all those other "strangers at the bedside." This has not happened.[10]

Perhaps because it has not, what empirical literature we have on IECs and their consultation function or the activities of individual consultants comes largely from those involved in their implementation. This literature stresses that most of those who have used consultative services have found the experience helpful, were satisfied with the results, and would request consultation again.[11] Of course, this does not tell us anything about the content of these consultations, the cases where consultation was appropriate but resisted (that is, satisfaction may be an artifact of self-selection) or even what exactly it was that created a "satisfying" consultation or "helpful" advice. The banality of this literature, which mimics social science in method and interpretation, is startling until one realizes that this is more an exhortatory than an informational literature. It exists to underscore that ethics committees are effective, deserve institutional resources, improve the quality of care, serve physician interests, and threaten no one. And all this may be so, but it would be nice to have some sociological discussion of the phenomenon.

Sociologically, Ethics Consultation May Not Be Such a Good Idea[12]

Until we have better data, we need to think about CEC theoretically. When we do so, a number of issues appear. All of them point to the inappropriateness of using IECs for ethical consultation. (Most of these remarks apply to individual ethics consultants as well, depending of course on the details of who is doing the consultation. To the extent that individual consultants are fellow clinicians, nurses, or physicians from within the organization, only the lack of a committee meeting itself makes any difference.) What is surprising is that whereas almost all these objections have been raised, occasionally forcefully, they have not been taken more seriously, and more has not been done either to see if the potential dangers occur or to guard against them. All speak to the difficulty of receiving an unbiased, independent reading of a case that is situated within an ongoing organizational context. (Of course, this assumes that what one wants is unbiased and independent and further suggests that medical consultations, such as those done by hematologists or infectious-disease subspecialists have this quality. Both assumptions can be questioned.) The very fact that some of these difficulties are both obvious and public yet disattended raises questions about whose interests IECs are designed to serve.

First, members of IECs, like members of most committees in most formal organizations, will have other roles to play in the organization. In most cases, these other roles are more important than voluntary committee service, which is more often than not uncompensated and unrewarding. Just because work is uncompensated and unrewarded does not mean workers will be slipshod. The fact that institutions can get their members to take on such thankless tasks seriously and work so hard at them is somewhat mysterious to us, all the more so when we are the ones donating the effort, losing the sleep, and struggling with issues that are unlikely to make us friends. Yet since IECs depend to a certain extent on exploited labor, the question always hangs in the air: How much effort is this worth? What is the personal price individuals are willing to pay to gear their ethical convictions into the world of cases that do not involve their patients?

With IECs, institutions can play upon the fact that those who toil in them with an interest in ethics are in the position of missionaries—they are bringing the word to colleagues who have not yet received it. Their own critique of care and their own sense of what is needed commits them to their work. The hospital, greedy organization that it is, can play upon these commitments and receive in turn a tremendous amount of unpaid labor. And here may lay the rub. As long as much of the labor is unpaid, it is devalued. Yet if the organization somehow were compelled to pay for the labor, it might decide it did not need it after all, but thank you anyway.

So ethicist is a role added to a primary-role system, which itself is coming under scrutiny to be more productive. In those other, more primary roles, committee members are likely to have dealings with the same colleagues whose ethical problems are now before them. In most situations, this is not a problem. Physicians understand that an ethics case consultation is not a trial, for they themselves may have initiated the consultation. Mature professionals recognize the difference between receiving advice and being judged.

Yet case consultations are not abstract affairs—they are not about words on a page or concepts in the abstract; they involve people in what is often a very closed world. Questions meant innocently to elicit information can bruise egos. Recommendations meant to resolve a stalemate can appear as an insult to one's judgment. The very fact that a dispute has reached an impasse such that those involved in it need avail themselves of a formally established procedure for dispute resolution can in itself be seen as an indictment of one's competence in the clinical arts or, worse, that one's behavior is seen by some as "unethical" and therefore a potential source of embarrassment. So, in the closed world of the tertiary care hospital, a world in which committee members may have very complex relations with those colleagues on whose case they are now consulting, an independent judgment unpolluted by all the other connections among co-workers in the organization should not be a taken-for-granted outcome. This one may be junior to that one and dependent on him or her for referrals. Or this one may be a rival with that one and wish for nothing so much as an occasion for public embarrassment. Committee members may have a variety of complex relations—friends, competitors, professional collaborators. In a word, they are colleagues. And when this consultation is over, when service on the committee is ended, they will continue to be colleagues coexisting in the same workspace.

The work of ethics committees then depends on individuals placed in dual relationships. This is of course true of other oversight committees in academic institutions, but it is a defect in them as well. Dual relationships are recognized by many professional codes of ethics as improper and banned. Committee members can recuse themselves if in their judgment the dual relationship poses a problem, but this places the burden on the individual member. It does not recognize how a complex structure of ongoing work relationships embeds the consultations of the hospital ethics committee in a continuous web of social interaction, most of which has nothing to do with this consultation but might be deeply affected by its outcome.[13]

If the image of the dual relationship seems overdrawn, perhaps we can appropriate another analogy to make the same point. In their fashion, ethics committee members are in a structural position similar to that of floor managers in industry.[14] The ethical standards and legal requirements for action can be thought of as management directives. The impasses, disputes, quandaries, and questions that come to committees for consultation can be thought of as problems on the line. The floor manager's job is to apply management's directives to line workers. This is not done without significant tension, compromise, and heartache, according to the ethnographers of the industrial workplace. Like the floor managers, members of the IEC are in the middle, subject to various and multitudinous forces—the pushes and pulls, strains and squeezes—which make it so hard to steer between the rocks and hard places of social life. It may also be the case that the farther members of IECs are from the everyday work of the hospital shop floor, the more devalued their consultative advice, suggestions, and recommendations are—just as industrial floor managers find their influence with workers wanes the closer they get to management. Moreover, just as floor managers are seen as ineffectual allies by workers when they are too distant from management to affect its directives, so may IEC members seem ineffective to those with whom they consult since committee members are constrained by legal rules and moral customs and are relatively powerless to change them. Further, to the degree their advice appears to suggest change in the handling of the case, they may, like floor managers who are punctilious about management's rules, be perceived as meddlers who do not have the interests of the workers at heart.

And, of course, suspicions and bad feelings may run in the other direction as well. In fact, they are much more likely to run that way. Behind almost every ethical problem that requires consultation, there is also a tangled social situation. Whether it involves the conflict of patients' families among themselves or with staff, or of staff among themselves, the kinds of situations that beget consultations are stressful.[15] In fact, if one just looks at those areas where health care is most problematic, it is hard to see how it could be otherwise. In many situations, consultation is a signal of a process stymied either by conflicted wills or deep moral qualms. In cases where families have conflict within themselves or with staff, there is bound to be some distrust of the hospital and its staff. Beyond that, the members of the ethics committee are likely to be strangers to families but not to hospital staff. There may be the sense that the consultation is just a charade to uphold the rationales, logic, and action that the family has had such problems with anyway. Procedurally, neither informality nor formality is likely to calm fears about fairness. Informality may lead to a sense of not being taken seriously, whereas formality can be seen to stack the deck in favor of organizational insiders who know the institution's ways. The point here is that if family members are allowed to present their story (some ethics committees do not allow this), when they look around the room they will see people who dress like, sound like, and look like the other staff who have given them such trouble. In such circumstances they may not feel like they have been given a fair hearing.[16]

Such feelings do indeed point to a real problem with CEC—how does the consultant or committee provide a hearing within the walls of the organization, yet provide and appear to provide an independent and even-handed reading of the situation?[17] This appearance of fairness is further compromised when CECs concern matters that have some bearing on the hospital and its standing. For example, in the late 1980s, surgeons at the University of Chicago began considering liver transplantation in children, using lobes from a living donor (the child's parent). The impetus was the shortage of cadaveric organs and the recognition that as many as a third of patients awaiting a liver die before an organ becomes available. This was the first such undertaking in the United States. Ethicists at the university began meeting with the involved surgeons and developed a proposal subsequently submitted to and accepted by the institution's IRB. The group displayed its reasoning in a report (Singer et al. 1989) that received widespread attention. A similar situation involved the University of Pittsburgh and its attempt to develop additional organ sources through the use of non–heart beating (that is, non–brain dead) organ donors (Frader 1993).

There was nothing egregiously wrong with the procedures or the justifications given by the committees approving them. Neither is at issue. Rather, the problem is the propriety of a committee ruling on a procedure in which so much is at stake institutionally. In cases of innovative medical action, where so much publicity is generated from being first, is there not tremendous pressure on organization members not to stand in the way? If all the boats rise with the tide, if organizational prestige is transferable to members of that organization, then there is something unrealistic about asking committee members to be the ethical arbiters of innovation. This is all the more so in tertiary care hospitals with their emphasis on research, innovations, and the clinical frontier.

In addition, the same point may cut the other way. Just as committee members may be chary of acting to slow innovation that promotes the good name of the institution, we may expect them to be equally chary of situations that could bring negative publicity to the institution. So, in cases where the chance of media spectacle is high and where attending physicians have decided that this game is not worth the candle, ethics committees may agree. Life is short. Committee members have other, more weighty responsibilities. The path of least resistance in such cases might be particularly attractive. How often consideration of the organization's good name comes into play is an empirical question, as are questions of how often such considerations skew decision making. Frequencies may be less important here than appearance. What is critical is that given their stake in the organization, ethics consultants and committee members have difficulty in making the claim that they are disinterested in that good name.

An additional problem presents itself when hospitals have very specific missions, besides the more general one of providing health care. For example, when hospitals are affiliated with religious communities, do IECs and consultants then have the additional responsibility of framing their reasoning in terms consistent with that religion's ethical standards? Are the ethics of a Catholic or Jewish hospital different from those of the larger, multicultural, pluralistic society of which they are a part (Loewy 1994)? If so, how far should these ethics apply to patients who are not members of the faithful? In public hospitals, what role do distributional questions play in weighing individual cases? In proprietary hospitals, are there specific obligations to consider shareholders' profits? In general, this may be seen as a problem of deciding how "universal" versus how "particularistic" CECs are intended to be. Denying the legitimacy of particularism seems an infringement on the prerogatives of individual organizations to chart their own destiny. Accepting it seems to deny patients the autonomy that CECs are intended to protect. On the other hand, affirming universalism appears to pretend an ethical certainty that we do not possess. Denying it accepts arbitrary choices and impositions of power that CECs would seem charged to avoid.

Finally, as Joel Frader (1992) has pointed out, there is something rather sociologically and politically naive in assuming that a committee ensures a decision representative of the community's will. The power inequities that characterize decision making outside the committee do not disappear simply by forming a committee. There is no guarantee that the more senior, the more powerful in the committee (or in the often less structured process used by individual consultants), will not dominate decision making. That is, disinterested decision making may be hostage to multiple considerations extraneous to the ethics of the case. Nurses may be dominated by physicians. Assistant professors may feel hostage to senior colleagues. This, like so many of the issues we have raised, is an empirical question; and like so many of the difficulties we have raised, it requires data before any judgment can be made.

Conclusion

As critics of health care, social scientists are a notoriously hard lot to please. For years they criticized mental hospitals as repressive places that stripped patients of their dignity, social identity, and civil rights while providing precious little in the way of therapy (see Goffman 1961 for the classic statement). When, partly in response to this critique, patients were deinstitutionalized, the critique was turned on its head, and social scientists found that patients in the community were degraded by the poor conditions in which they lived, harmed by overmedication, and deprived of dignity, social worth, and autonomy.

For years social scientists critiqued a fee-for-service system that was said to provide powerful incentives for unnecessary treatment, to create fee barriers limiting access to necessary care, and to undermine the professional integrity of physicians overly aware of their economic self-interest (see Freidson 1970 for the classic statement). Now, when, in part as a response to this critique, managed care regimes have been instituted, we have turned this critique on its head. Prepaid capitated health care is said to discourage needed services, to create barriers of access because of the reluctance to enroll those who are in less than perfect health or have actuarial risks, and to undermine the professional integrity of physicians overly aware of their self-interest (Rodwin 1993 provides a useful overview).

For years social scientists critiqued physicians for their policies of information control. Physicians were said to control tightly what information was passed to patients, to magnify clinical uncertainty, and in general to limit autonomy by preventing patients and their family access to necessary information (Quint 1967; Davis 1963; Glaser and Strauss 1965, 1967, 1968; Strauss 1970). Often such policies were justified as a way of minimizing the emotional distress associated with illness. In operation they were said to frustrate patients' ability to provide informed consent for treatment. With more muscular notions of patients' rights and informed consent, physicians' practices changed. Now they were criticized for overwhelming patients with technical information, not providing enough emotional support to patients, and limiting their role responsibilities to the narrowest possible technical domain. No sooner than the suggestions of critics of health care are implemented, then those same critics carp at the unintended consequences of the planned social change. Under such conditions we might expect that those who, with the best of intentions, try to improve the quality of health care through ethics consultation may experience substantial frustration.

We have identified the sociological currents that run through CECs—the next step is for social scientists to begin watching CECs work, attending to these sociological dimensions. Only then will we discover how CECs extend, limit, or otherwise redirect medical power.

References

Anspach, Renee R. 1993. *Deciding who lives: Fateful choices in the intensive-care nursery.* Berkeley: University of California Press.

Barber, Bernard, et al. 1973. *Research on human subjects: Problems of social control in medical experimentation.* New York: Sage.

Bloom, Bernard S., and Osler L. Peterson. 1973. End results, cost and productivity of coronary-care units. *New England Journal of Medicine* 288: 72–8.

Bosk, Charles L. 1992. *All God's mistakes: Genetic counseling in a pediatric hospital.* Chicago: University of Chicago Press.

Chambliss, Daniel F. 1993. Is bioethics irrelevant? *Contemporary Sociology* 22(5): 649–52.

———. 1996. *Beyond caring: Hospitals, nurses, and the social organization of ethics.* Chicago: University of Chicago Press.

Cransford, Ronald E., and A. Edward Doudera. 1984. The emergence of institutional ethics committees. *Law Medicine & Health Care* 12(1): 13–20.

Crigger, Bette Jane. 1995. Bioethnography: Fieldwork in the lands of medical ethics. *Medical Anthropology Quarterly,* n.s., 9(3): 400–17.

Danis, Marion, Leslie I. Southerland, Joanne M. Garrett, et al. 1991. A prospective study of advance directives for life-sustaining care. *New England Journal of Medicine* 324: 882–8.

Davis, Fred. 1963. *Passage through crisis: Polio victims and their families.* Indianapolis: Bobbs-Merrill.

DeVries, Raymond G. 1995. Toward a sociology of bioethics. *Qualitative Sociology* 18(1): 119–28.

Duff, Raymond S., and A. G. M. Campbell. 1973. Moral and ethical dilemmas in the special-care nursery. *New England Journal of Medicine* 289(17): 890–4.

Fisher, Bernard, Madeline Bauer, Richard Margolesse, et al. 1985. Five-year results of a randomized clinical trial comparing total mastectomy and segmental mastectomy with or without radiation in the treatment of breast cancer. *New England Journal of Medicine* 312: 665–73.

Fleetwood, Janet E., Robert M. Arnold, and Richard J. Baron. 1989. Giving answers or raising questions? The problematic role of institutional ethics committees. *Journal of Medical Ethics* 15: 137–42.

Fleetwood, Janet, and Stephanie S. Unger. 1994. Institutional ethics committees and the shield of immunity. *Annals of Internal Medicine* 120: 320–5.

Fletcher, John C., Norman Quist, and Albert R. Jonsen. 1989. Ethics consultation in health care: Rationale and history. In *Ethics Consultation in Health Care,* edited by John C. Fletcher, Norman Quist, and Albert R. Jonsen. Ann Arbor, Mich.: Health Administration Press.

Fox, Renée C. 1989. The sociology of bioethics. In *The sociology of medicine: A participant observer's view.* Englewood Cliffs, N.J.: Prentice Hall.

Fox, Renée C., and Judith P. Swazey. 1974. *The courage to fail: A social view of organ transplantation and dialysis.* Chicago: University of Chicago Press.

———. 1992. *Spare parts: Organ replacement in American society.* New York: Oxford University Press.

Frader, Joel E. 1992. Political and interpersonal aspects of ethics consultation. *Theoretical Medicine* 13: 31–44.

———. 1993. Non-heart-beating organ donation: Personal and institutional conflicts of interest. *Kennedy Institute of Ethics Journal* 3(2): 189–98.

Frank, Arthur W. 1995. *The wounded storyteller: Body, illness, and ethics.* Chicago: University of Chicago Press.

Freidson, Eliot. 1970. *Profession of medicine: A study of the sociology of applied knowledge.* New York: Harper & Row.

Glaser, Barney G., and Anselm L. Strauss. 1965. *Awareness of dying.* Chicago: Aldine.

———. 1967. *The discovery of grounded theory; Strategies for qualitative research.* Chicago: Aldine.

———. 1968. *Time for dying.* Chicago: Aldine.

Goffman, Erving. 1961. *Asylums, essays on the social situation of mental patients and other inmates.* Garden City, N.Y: Anchor Books.

Gray, Bradford H. 1975. *Human subjects in medical experimentation: A sociological study of the conduct and regulation of clinical research.* New York: Wiley.

Hare, Jan, Clara Pratt, and Carrie Nelson. 1992. Agreement between patients and their self-selected surrogates on difficult medical decisions. *Archives of Internal Medicine* 152: 1049–54.

Hess, Orvan W. 1980. Impact of electronic fetal monitoring on obstetric management. *Journal of the American Medical Association* 244: 682–6.

La Puma, John. 1987. Consultations in clinical ethics—issues and questions in 27 cases. *Western Journal of Medicine* 146: 633–7.

La Puma, John, and David L. Schiedermayer. 1991. Ethics consultation: Skills, roles, and training. *Annals of Internal Medicine* 114: 155–60.

La Puma, John, Carol B. Stocking, Marc D. Silverstein, et al. 1988. An ethics consultation service in a teaching hospital: Utilization and evaluation. *Journal of the American Medical Association* 260: 808–11.

La Puma, John, Carol B. Stocking, Cheryl M. Darling, and Mark Siegler. 1992. Community hospital ethics consultation: Evaluation and comparison with a university hospital service. *American Journal of Medicine* 92: 346–51.

Levine, Murray. 1983. IRB review as a "cooling out device." *IRB: A Review of Human Subjects* 5(4): 8–9.

Lo, Bernard. 1987. Behind closed doors: Promises and pitfalls of ethics committees. *New England Journal of Medicine* 317: 46–50.

Loewy, Erich. 1994. Institutional morality, authority, and ethics committees: How far should respect for institutional morality go? *Cambridge Quarterly of Healthcare Ethics* 3(4): 578–84.

McClung, John A., Russel S. Kamer, Margaret DeLuca, and Harlan J. Barber. 1996. Evaluation, of a medical ethics consultation service: Opinions of patients and health care providers. *American Journal of Medicine* 100: 456–60.

McCrary, S. Van, and Jeffery R. Botkin. 1989. Hospital policy on advance directives: Do institutions ask patients about living wills? *Journal of the American Medical Association* 262: 2411–4.

Moreno, Jonathan D. 1995. *Deciding together: Bioethics and moral consensus.* New York: Oxford University Press.

Nelson, Karin B., James M. Dambrosia, Tricia Y. Ting, and Judith K. Grether. 1996. Uncertain value of electronic fetal monitoring in predicting cerebral palsy. *New England Journal of Medicine* 334: 613–18.

Paris, John J., Robert K. Crone, and Frank Reardon. 1990. Physicians' refusal of requested treatment: The case of Baby L. *New England Journal of Medicine* 322: 1012–5.

Paris, John J., Michael D. Schreiber, Mindy Statter, et al. 1993. Beyond autonomy—physicians' refusal to use life-prolonging extracorporeal membrane oxygenation. *New England Journal of Medicine* 329: 354–7.

Perkins, Henry S., and Bonnie S. Saathoff. 1988. Impact of medical ethics consultations on physicians: An exploratory study. *American Journal of Medicine* 85: 761–5.

Quint, Jeanne C: 1967. *The nurse and the dying patient.* New York: Macmillan.

Robertson, John A., and Norman Fost. 1976. Passive euthanasia of defective newborns: Legal considerations. *Journal of Pediatrics* 88: 883–7.

Rodwin, Marc A. 1993. *Medicine, money, and morals: Physicians' conflicts of interest.* New York: Oxford University Press.

Ross, Judith Wilson. 1986. *Handbook for hospital ethics committees.* Chicago: American Hospital Publishing.

Rothenberg, Leslie Steven. 1989. Clinical ethicists and hospital ethics consultants: The nature of the "clinical" role. In *Ethics consultation in health care,* edited by John C. Fletcher, Norman Quist, and Albert R. Jonsen. Ann Arbor, Mich.: Health Administration Press.

Scofield, Giles R. 1993. Ethics consultation: The least dangerous profession? *Cambridge Quarterly of Healthcare Ethics* 2: 417–26.

Sehgal, Aswini, Alison Galbraith, Margaret Chesney, et al. 1992. How strictly do dialysis patients want their advance directives followed? *Journal of the American Medical Association* 267: 59–63.

Singer, Peter A., Mark Siegler, Peter F. Whitington, et al. 1989. Ethics of liver transplantation with living donors. *New England Journal of Medicine* 321: 620–2.

Stelter, Keith L., Barbara A. Elliott, and Candace A. Bruno. 1992. Living will completion in older adults. *Archives of Internal Medicine* 152: 954–9.

Strauss, Anselm L., ed. 1970. *Where medicine fails*. Chicago: Aldine.

Teel, Karen. 1975. The physician's dilemma: A doctor's view: What the law should be. *Baylor Law Review* 27 (winter): 6, 8–10.

Tomlinson, Tom, Kenneth Howe, Mark Notman, and Diane Rossmiller. 1990. An empirical study of proxy consent for elderly persons. *Gerontologist* 30: 54–64.

Ulhmann, Richard F., Robert A. Pearlman, and Kevin C. Cain. 1988. Physicians' and spouses' predictions of elderly patients' resuscitation preferences. *Journal of Gerontology* 43: M115–21.

Wertz, Dorothy C., James R. Sorenson, and Timothy C. Heeren. 1988. "Can't get no (dis)satisfaction": Professional satisfaction with professional-client encounters. *Work and Occupations* 15: 36–54.

Zaner, Richard M. 1993. Voices and time: The venture of clinical ethics. *Journal of Medicine and Philosophy* 18: 9–31.

Zussman, Robert 1992. *Intensive care: Medical ethics and the medical profession*. Chicago: University of Chicago Press.

Zweibel, Nancy R., and Christine K. Cassel. 1989. Treatment choices at the end of life: A comparison of decisions by older patients and their physician-selected proxies. *Gerontologist* 29: 615–21.

Notes

1. This is not the place to assess how well IRBs have succeeded at the tasks assigned them. Suffice it to say that, almost simultaneously with the establishment of federal standards, there was the establishment of a research literature that looked critically at the operation of IRBs. Early examples included Barber et al. (1973) and Gray (1975). It is worth noting that there has been little addition to that literature since those early days. We really don't have much idea whether contemporary IRBs in fact do what they were set up to accomplish.

   At the same time, to document compliance with federal regulations, the administrative functions of both hospital and university research needed to be expanded. This was matched by the formation and growth of the federal Office for the Protection from Research Risk (OPRR) to oversee the IRB function and a similar office in the Food and Drug Administration to oversee that agency's rules about the investigation of drugs and devices. In 1979 a nongovernmental agency, the Hastings Center, introduced *IRB*, a journal that serves as a forum for the discussion of intellectual and administrative issues regarding human research subjects.

2. A recent treatise by Moreno (1995), a philosopher, on efforts to achieve consensus in bioethics provides a more comprehensive, if also idiosyncratic, historical account of the rise of ethics committees. Moreno notes that committees, beginning in the 1920s and 1930s, often deliberated on which mentally handicapped persons would have sterilization procedures. Somewhat later, small committees stood in judgment over which women would have abortions prior to the *Roe v. Wade* decision by the U.S. Supreme Court.

3. When asking CLB to serve on this panel, whose official title is the SHHV-SBC Task Force on Standards for Bioethics Consultation, the task force co-director who issued the invitation made it clear that it was CLB's lack of involvement in and knowledge about ethics consultation that made him an attractive potential member. The co-director was looking for an "outsider who knew something about professionalization." Given that so many fit this description, CLB was flattered to be asked. It should probably be mentioned as well that the other of us (JF), though not a task force member, drafted the original submission to the foundation pointing out the need for such a panel.

4. A peculiar feature of this point is that it is valid, even though as we will argue in the text, it is difficult to specify exactly what the content of that expertise is or what the nature of those skills are. In any case, it is not so clear that the purpose of the hospital ethics committee is to provide an expert opinion. When opinions are called for, when advice is sought, its expertness in these cases might not be its most important quality. Again, we will deal with this point in the text as well.

5. Anspach (1993) has pointed out how physicians psychologize dissent among the families of children in neonatal intensive care units. Parents who disagree—rather than being seen as having their reasons, their values, and their life-plans—are seen as disturbed, subjects for psychological services. Bosk (1992) found that genetic counselors were used in much the same way. Emotional and ethical work were split off from the more technical aspects of doctoring. This work was then turfed to genetic counselors. But Anspach and Bosk both did their fieldwork before the current institutionalization of ethics in the hospital. We are suggesting that the ethics committee may now be used in much the same way.

6. Many of these points apply to ethics consultation when done by individuals in the role of ethicist, as well as when they are functioning in committees. Others—those specifically about committee dynamics—do not.

7. Our caution here refers primarily to recently published results of the SUP-PORT project. That research carefully documented the lack of impact on end-of-life medical decisions in tertiary intensive care units despite detailed feedback to clinicians about the preferences and experience, especially pain and suffering, of the critically ill patients.

8. As noted before, there is an interesting contrast here to the response of sociologists to informed consent regulations. Here researchers first documented processes that made the case for fuller communication and then began almost immediately looking at the impact of new regulations. We might wonder why one change generated a response among researchers while the other did not.

9. This point is worth belaboring with some theory. The process is sociologically interesting whichever metaphorical perspective one adopts for looking at professionals. Whether describing a Hughesian "struggle for license and mandate"; a Bucherian and Straussian "shared community of identity and fate"; a Sarfitti–Larsonian "project"; a Parsonsian adoption of "fiduciary responsibility"; an Abbotian "jurisdictional struggle"; or a Freidsonian "professional dominance"—the empirical phenomenon of a new area of responsibility in partly the same old and partly new hands is a phenomenon of intrinsic empirical interest. The fact that one both so visible and so adaptable to one's favorite propositions about professions is at the same time so ignored is difficult to explain.

10. We will not speculate much here about why this has not occurred, however tempted we are. We cannot resist the opportunity to suggest that one reason for our lack of interest may itself be a latent consequence of a sociological tendency to think in terms of the manifest and the latent. Actually, these days we use other terms not so loaded with the connotations of a discarded functionalism. We write of the implicit and the explicit, the tacit and the taken for granted, the public and the private, the revealed and the hidden, the surface and the deep structure, the *parole* and the *langue*—whatever. However we label the dichotomy, the underlying conceptual operations are the same—scratch surface explanations deep enough and we find self-interest. It may be that we sociologists have not looked at the new occupation of ethicist and the new practices of ethical consultation because we are already certain of their meaning—they are and can be nothing more than an attempt to preserve professional power by internalizing a critique and thereby disarming it. In this line of thinking, IECs are simply a way of silencing resistance and challenges to medical authority by taking charge of the dispute process and professionalizing it. In this light, it is again worth noting the number of physician-ethicists who claim that medical ethicists who consult must also be physicians.

11. It is worth noting here that in another context, Wertz, Sorenson, and Heeren (1988) were puzzled by their inability to discover any dissatisfaction in patient surveys of genetic counselors. It may be that dissatisfaction is hard to elicit—although this is a conclusion that rings false to us, subjected as we are to regular student evaluations. An alternative explanation is that satisfaction or dissatisfaction is relative to expectations. So, if expectations are sufficiently negative and if nothing untoward results, then users of a service may report satisfaction. The point to be stressed is that satisfaction does not stand alone with some pristine meaning. Rather, we need to know as well why an encounter was satisfying and what was satisfying about it. For example, we are satisfied with our dentist every time we go and do not need a root canal. This satisfaction has little to do with the service rendered and is clearly inappropriate as a proxy measure for that service's quality.

12. It is only fair to inform the reader that one of the authors (JF) actually engages in the practice of clinical ethics consultation and has been a member of the board of directors of the national organization promoting such activity. The reader will have to decide if or how this confuses the picture sketched herein.

13. One might object that this is really an empirical, not a theoretical, point. Rather than cast general aspersions, we should give specific examples. Of course, specific examples require just that kind of research that we argued is so necessary. Our own experience in academic environments suggests that it is possible for other agendas to temper ethical commitments, to avoid confrontation, or to build alliances and trust.

14. Right here we are engaging in a rather straightforward Hughesian analysis of the workplace, trying to find the dilemmas of high-status work in a less exalted workplace.

15. Once again, we must note that there is a tendency to think about ethics problems as representing conflict, an inability of the parties involved to reach a moral consensus. Though convenient, such language obscures that even when there is agreement among the parties, even when they have reached consensus, an ethics consult may be needed. The parties may need to reassure each other that what they wish to do is both morally acceptable and socially feasible. The image of moral conflict among the parties has the defect of suggesting that one is right (and hence ethical and moral) while the other is wrong (and hence, at least in this instance, a moral reprobate). It ignores the way ethical conflict involves opposing rights that then need to be balanced, mediated, or compromised. A second problem of the notion of ethical conflict with resolution by committee deliberation is that it reinforces an adversarial, judicial perspective and a language of rights. Neither is the only way nor may either be the best way to think about ethical issues. Finally, an image of ethics problems as conflict on the shop floor overlooks how much that parties agree to may be nonetheless ethically problematic.

    Two interrelated phenomena are at work in the conflict imagery. First, there is a tendency to ethicize problems related to social structure. This transforms issues of power and authority—and more recently, economics—into issues of principle—generally, autonomy, beneficence, nonmalfeasance, and justice. This is a particularly effective strategy for those with lesser power. It is a strategy of empowerment that helps level the playing field.

    Second, once structural problems have been turned into ethical problems, there is a social tendency to turn them into legal ones. This move places an emphasis on contending parties, formal rules of procedure (including what things to count as evidence for propositions), and then justifications for action in terms of principles. The emphasis here becomes not just this case but all cases that could arise in the future and would be like this case. The legalism may be extremely ad hoc—that is, difficult consultations create the need for procedures that may fall into disuse until the next difficult or controversial case, at which point the procedures may be revised.

16. What is at issue here is not the actual fairness or the reasonableness of consultative advice (if in fact such advice and recommendations are even communicated to families). Both may be impeccable, as may be the motivations and intent of committee members. What is at issue is, when those from lay culture contend with those from the professional culture of the hospital, nothing short of total acquiescence of those in authority can convince the family that they really were taken seriously.

17. We have here used the circumlocution "provide and appear to provide" since both are so important to the appearance of justice. We have no doubt that committees make their best efforts to render the best judgments possible. But with the growing divide between professional culture and lay culture, with the professionalization of the ethics function, and with the bureaucratization and routinization of ethical conflicts, it seems quite possible that, however just the actual reasoning of committees or consultants, the appearance of justice will be wanting.

FOUR

Margin of Error

THE SOCIOLOGY OF ETHICS CONSULTATION

Introduction

The title of this chapter is divided by a colon. The first three words of that title, "Margin of Error," appear to the left of the colon and are an implied question, a world of interpretive possibilities suggested by a phrase evocative in its ambiguity. This world is erased by the more exacting semantic construction that appears to the right of the colon in the original working title: "The Nature, Inevitability, and Ethics of Mistakes in Medicine and Bioethics Consultation." The title is a binary opposition. The left is the raw; the wild; the animal; the sacred; the dark; and, of course the left. The right is the cooked; the tamed; the human; the profane; the light; and, of course, the right.

The right, being both the side that it is and the part of the opposition that it expresses is capable of much further subdivision. The disciplined and disciplinary half of the colonic divide, it represents our scientific, theological, and philosophic understanding. It is the side in which the terms *margin* and *error* come to have operational definitions both for those such as ethics consultants or clinical ethicists who need to act in situations of risky choice

Chapter 4 was originally published as "Margin of Error: The Sociology of Ethics Consultation," in *Margin of Error: The Nature, Inevitability, and Ethics of Error in Biomedical and Ethics Consultation,* ed. S. Rubin and L. Zoloth-Dorff. (University Press of America, Spring 2000).

where help is needed and for those who are trying to make sense out of these newly specialized and socially visible activities that we call clinical ethics consultation.

The tension of this chapter is that the right side of the title seeks to make sense of the left, but the left always has an incalculable element of terrifying mystery and awesome power. When we cross the divide of the colon—when we transform error into mistake—we perform an important collective ritual affirming, denying, and thereby neutralizing that mystery and power that resides leftwards of the colon. In this ritual, whatever form it takes, we press for and provide a social accounting for the error. This social accounting assigns to each error a cause, identifies warning signals to prevent such errors in the future, provides ground rules for understanding and action the next time, and reaffirms first principles for pressing on with the enterprise now that we have addressed the problem.

Untamed error exists as the Kennedy assassination; the launch of the Challenger and its subsequent explosion; the fiery crash of TWA Flight 800; the immolation of the Branch Davidian compound; the assault of Rodney King by Los Angeles police officers; and, closer to my home, the bombing by the Philadelphia police of the MOVE headquarters or the explosive collision of U.S. Senator John Heinz's private jet and a helicopter over a schoolyard during lunch recess. All of these are examples of errors in their pure state. Errors are, above all, a breakdown in the normal organization of social life as a practical accomplishment, an ongoing natural order within a meaningful world. Many of the above errors were all the more threatening to our sense of how the world works by the fact of their being captured on film or tape for endless playing and replaying. Each new viewing raises again the fundamental question: How could this happen? At the same time, each reviewing deadens our collective horror and wonder of the world gone awry. Public disaster and the implications it carries of human failing so ruptures our taken-for-granted sense of how the world works—our normal expectations—that a collective search for the explanation of error is necessary.

These public errors have their shocking properties removed through a public process that turns the incomprehensible mishap into a mistake that had its reasons. These reasons allow blame to be assigned to individuals and the more structural, global implications of error to be evaded. With serious error—undeniable breaches to the normal order—there is something like a ritual order for the restoration of the everyday: an impartial blue-ribbon panel is set up to investigate the rending of normal expectations, the error. Panels are comprised of members selected for disciplinary or technical expertise, demographic diversity, and political centrality. Panels then find a set of specific reasons to explain this error in the natural order; they tame error by labeling and categorizing the mistakes that allowed it to occur, reducing the intrinsic tragedy of error to a set of mere miscalculations avoidable in the future. Panels sometimes find that their pronouncements are met with profound skepticism in some quarters. Error is not so easily tamed as the right side of its existence likes to pretend; those who read left-sided meanings into error's inevitable existence resist official normalizing accounts. The political dexterity needed to turn errors into mistakes is seen as a sinister plot by those who find in errors other, more primordial meanings.

But, error in medicine and bioethics consultation is surely different from the kind of error that results in socially visible catastrophe. The Challenger, TWA Flight 800, Pan Am Flight 104, Bhopal, Chernobyl, Three Mile Island—their occurrence and the subsequent need to account for that existential fact—these surely share few characteristics with the errors of medicine and bioethics consultation. At the surface, the denial of any commonalities seems sensible. Socially visible errors are accounted for in and with very public processes; public hearings, testimonials, and reports provide the democratic transparency of a public inquiry, the social openness of a visible collective grappling with human failure, and the public judgment of a final report.

Error in medicine and bioethics consultation occurs in a different social space entirely. Social accounts for error are certainly, on occasion, necessary. But errors, for the most part, are internalized by the provider organization, however this is defined, or the appropriate operating unit of the organization identified as responsible for that error. In the socially visible error of the public catastrophe, the fact of error is inescapable. An analysis of decision making will lead back to causes and the identification of responsible parties. In the arena of medicine, the process of identifying and accounting for mistakes is very different. Whether error, in fact, occurred is often hotly contested. Who is the responsible agent is also a source of debate without resolution. Even when errors are acknowledged, there is still very rarely public reporting of specific incidents. Rarer still is the public linking of individuals with particular mistakes. This is to say the social accounting system in medicine is much more private. The difference in the type of event that sparks an inquiry and the processes then used to account for that error suggests that there is little to learn by comparing publicly visible catastrophe to the more quiet disaster of medicine and bioethics consultation. Practically speaking, the margin of error in medicine and bioethics is so wide that we can live happily on the right side of the colon of this volume's title. This essay questions that assumption by surveying what we know of medical error in the context of what we know about public catastrophe. What we learn from supplementing one perspective on error and mistakes with the other is then applied to discuss error and mistakes in bioethics consultations.

Two Sociologies of Error

Error and the social accounts offered to explain it are relatively underdeveloped domains within sociology. Sociological theory has more often concentrated on explaining success. In many ways our theories echo a public ideology or American civil religion; the accent is on progress, development, and programmatic action to overcome obstacles and barriers to social achievement. Despite the minimal emphasis on how errors are identified, categorized, understood, and managed, two disparate, albeit complementary perspectives have emerged for viewing error. One perspective concentrates on organizational features of error; the other focuses on emergent understandings in the everyday life of the work group.

THE ORGANIZATION OF NORMAL ERROR

Charles Perrow is a leading proponent of the organizational approach to error.[1] He contends that modern technological systems are error prone and that we should think of certain catastrophes, such as mishaps at nuclear power plants, as "normal accidents." For Perrow, certain accidents are not produced by individual human failings—what he call the "ubiquitous operator error." Rather, certain catastrophes are an inevitable result of features embedded in many enterprises of the modern world. The two features most important to the production of normal accidents are interactive complexity and tight coupling; that is, each system component is itself intrinsically complicated at the same time that each component part's performance affects the functioning of other system components. As a result, errors ramify through systems, creating large catastrophes. This is simply a fact of life for many of our complex technological undertakings. Or, as Perrow says: "If interactive complexity and tight coupling—system characteristics—inevitably will produce an accident, I believe we are justified in calling it a *normal accident* or *system accident*. The odd term *normal accident* is meant to signal that, given the system characteristics, multiple and unexpected interactions of failure are inevitable. This is an expression of an integral part of the system, not a statement of frequency."[2]

We cannot, says Perrow, prevent normal accidents by simply building more elaborate warning and backup safety systems. These systems add to the complexity and tight coupling of the organization of the original enterprise. They become as likely to malfunction as any other part of the system. Safety devices then multiply the possibilities for normal error. Any reduction in the probability of error is more than offset by the new component with its own unique possibility for failing and sending mistaken signals to other components of the system. Perrow's survey of normal accidents in high-risk systems is a mind-numbing catalogue of all the ways a concern for safety creates complacency, misperception, or misjudgment in the face of alarming dangers. For Perrow, what is needed is not merely better safety systems or more diligence, for the marginal gain from these is just too unpredictable. What is needed is better wisdom about which high-risk technologies to encourage and which to abandon.

The most extensive empirical treatment of a normal accident is Diane Vaughan's *The Challenger Launch Decision*.[3] To watch, as a nation of schoolchildren did, the technological pomp and ceremony surrounding this launch (which featured Christa McAuliffe, the nation's first teacher-astronaut shuttle passenger), then witness the explosion of the spacecraft in real time, watch the visible, smoke-flumed pieces of wreckage drop into the ocean, and listen to startled newscasters search for adequate words to describe and explain what happened, was to experience firsthand the power, horror, and mystery of error on the left side of our chapter's title. Vaughan's historical ethnography accomplishes two separate explanatory tasks.

First Vaughan shows the social and organizational work needed to remove the horror, mystery, and power of the visual images of original error—to normalize the explosion as a "deviant outcome," one not rooted in the organizational culture of the National Aeronautics and Space Administration (NASA) and private aerospace contractors like Morton-Thiokol. To do this, Vaughan analyzes how the official "Rogers Commission" report constructed an explanation that emphasized the decision to launch as a mistake that ignored previous warnings that something was amiss with the O-rings. The official understanding of the event lays the blame at a few reckless individuals who foolishly overrode the evidence of past performance and the expertise of fearful engineers. This scripting of the final report satisfies certain cultural requirements for adequate social accounting for error by locating the source of the disaster, demonstrating how far that source was from our normal expectations, and underlining how what was learned in analyzing this disaster will prevent its recurrence in the future.

Second, and more importantly, Vaughan demonstrates that the official account of the decision to launch the Challenger is a "just-so" song we whistle to ourselves as we walk alone through the graveyards of high-risk technologies at night. The problem with the official account is that it is inaccurate. In Vaughan's judgment, the decision to launch the Challenger was not the result of deviant behavior by NASA personnel. On the contrary, the decision was the result of sets of interacting workers following work group norms that had developed over time. The most important of these were the normalization of deviant performance of the O-rings over several flights; a production culture that had made accommodations to the built-in budgetary constraints of the shuttle program; and patterns of communication between operating units of the launch team that created a structure of secrecy as an artifact of bureaucratic reporting requirements. Information was passed up the organization but not necessarily shared between parallel subunits. This pattern of communication brought into being what David Matza, in the far different context of explaining juvenile delinquency, identified as zones of "pluralistic ignorance."[4] Those with doubts and misgivings were not in a position where they could share their thoughts and misgivings with anyone but their organizational superiors. The opportunities for "private troubles" to escalate into "public issues" were constricted as a result.

If it does nothing else, this abbreviated account of normal accidents underscores that the work place of the tertiary-care hospital shares features with workplaces said to be most typical of those where normal accidents occur. There is interactive complexity and tight coupling. Clinical emergencies that demand action before information is complete are commonplace. There are laboratory tests and bedside monitoring units that perform just as erratically as O-rings. Work groups develop a production culture where economic constraint is a brutal fact of any calculation of what to do. Patterns of everyday interaction create zones of pluralistic ignorance between operating units of the organization. As a raw fact of organizational life, there is an irreducible structure of secrecy in tertiary care that is a contributing factor to much of the normal error that occurs. Although normal errors have tragic consequences, although they are all too costly and frequent, and although efforts to reduce such errors are necessary, once a basic investment in safety is made, further investment is likely to provide disappointing marginal gains. Some activities such as space travel or healthcare, activities premised on highly sophisticated technological processes, are "error-ridden."

THE CULTURE AND PRODUCTION OF ERROR ON THE SHOP FLOOR

The organizational approach sees error as one of the normal products of task organization. The second approach in the sociology of error begins where the organizational approach leaves off. Starting with the assumption that work is "error-ridden," this second perspective revolves around the culture and production of error on the shop floor. Some of the first studies of error are literally of shop floors: production crews in the aircraft industry,[5] workers in a machine shop,[6] street-level bureaucrats,[7] or managers in an industrial plant.[8] However, the most sustained treatment of workplace error concentrates on the shop floor of the academic hospital.

The classic orienting statement for understanding medical error is Everett C. Hughes's essay "Mistakes at Work."[9] For Hughes, all work can be categorized as either routines or emergencies. Routines, when routinely attended to with success, reinforce a sense of mastery. Routines that do not yield success create emergencies. Emergencies, when handled with aplomb, create routines and thereby reestablish a sense of competence and mastery. Emergencies that spiral out of control create the sense that a culpable error or mistake was made, and that sense is a threat to the integrity of the work activity. Mistakes and errors create the impression that those involved do not know what they are doing. Hughes suggests that we can create a calculus for mistakes and errors out of the experience of the worker and the routineness of the task.

Because academic hospitals often involve front-line workers (students and residents) who may have little experience, and because the clinical problems encountered there are often very far from routine on any standard index, we might expect to find a fair number of mistakes and errors. But, says Hughes, hospital work is organized in such a way as both to control and limit the actual occurrence of mistakes and to filter out any recognition of individual responsibility or accountability for mistakes. Hughes describes the organization of hospital work as a set of "risk-sharing" and "guilt-shifting" devices that make it difficult to say if or exactly where in the chain of events the error or mistake occurred. These work practices include supervision, consultation, cross-coverage, and case conferences. All of these devices make it harder to see individual mistakes. A course of action is not any one individual's property or agency, but rather it is shared within a community of fellow workers who second decisions all along the way. For Hughes errors are normal, and there is an elaborated social division of labor that keeps errors and mistakes from coming plainly into view. In his recent discussions of training for certainty, Paul Atkinson has clearly restated this position and given it greater empirical specificity.[10] Paget[11] and West[12] have provided two leading accounts detailing how mistakes are embedded in the everyday order and language of the group. The old folk adage, "Doctors bury their mistakes," describes better the social process that surrounds mistakes and errors than it does the literal fate of patients. Not all mistakes are so meaningful, so fateful.

Even so, not all medical mistakes can be buried. Some outcomes of care raise a strong, if rebuttable, presumption that a serious error has occurred. These outcomes are public and visible, as are the social accounting practices and collective rituals employed to rebut the more serious implications of fateful error. Light extends Hughes's discussion of mistakes at work by looking at the type of negative outcome that is not so easily folded into the life of the group, not so easily hidden from view.[13] The error that Light examines is suicide from the perspective of the treating physician (a resident) and the work group (the ward and the training program). His account of a suicide review sounds a number of important points for our understanding of mistakes at work and recognizes suicide review as a workplace ritual that serves a number of group needs. First, the artful discussion of the case models professional standards at precisely the moment the event being reviewed makes a mockery of claims to competent practice. Second, the faults of the individual therapist in handling the case are pointed out in such a gentle way as to suggest that these misjudgments could (indeed, would) have been made by anyone—that the errors involved were inevitable and unavoidable; hence, the errors need not weigh too heavily on the head of the therapist or the supervisor. And third, the lessons of the case taken away from the review, in Light's words, provide "a reaffirmation of how fine psychiatry is; for in its darkest hour, a clear lesson can be drawn by a model of the profession (the reviewer)."[14] Errors are inevitable and unfortunate. But they also serve as an occasion for reviewing behavior and for correcting faulty practice. However, as Light points out, the perforce adhoc and episodic nature of suicide review prevents us from making broad generalizations about the lessons from suicides.

It is on the generalizable dimensions of the social accounting for error that I concentrate in *Forgive and Remember: Managing Medical Failure*.[15] This ethnographic study examines how surgical residents learn to separate blameless error from blameworthy mistakes in the course of their training. Errors appear blameless, by and large, if they are seen as part of the normal learning process. Inexperienced residents are expected to make some technical or judgmental mistakes. These errors are considered a normal consequence of providing opportunities to the unpracticed. Such difficulties have the following characteristics: the resident quickly recognizes the problem; the resident seeks appropriate help for it; the resident learns a "lesson" from the entire incident; and the resident does not repeat that mistake during the rotation. These are normal errors; like Perrow's normal accidents that are built into the system of technology, these are built into the system of training. These normal errors allow the attending physician and resident to take the role of teacher and student, respectively. Attending physicians say they "forgive and remember" the normal errors of their residents. They forgive because such errors are inevitable in a field like surgery. They remember just in case such errors are repeated, become part of a pattern, and thereby indicate that something in addition to the normal fallibility of a diligent and scrupulous resident is causing these errors.

If error that can be seen as part of the educational process is seen as both normal and blameless, then errors are blameworthy when the reading of events makes it difficult to sustain a claim that the resident acted in good faith. Errors are blameworthy when they involve normative breaches—that is, when they break universal rules about how a responsible doctor acts. Also blameworthy are quasi-normative breaches or the failure to abide by an attending physician's cherished but often idiosyncratic way of doing things. A source of great confusion to residents is the fact that attending physicians treat breaches of their personal rules as seriously as they do breaches of universal rules. Hence residents' views of egregious errors are often at odds with those of attending physicians, especially if the attending physicians have confused their personal preferences with the moral order. Difficulties likely to be coded as normative have the following characteristics: the resident failed to recognize problems sufficiently early or attempted to cover them up; the resident failed to seek appropriate help; the resident failed to improve his or her performance over successive trials; and the resident made the same mistake on repeated occasions. These errors are not seen as a normal part of the educational process, but rather they signal that a resident lacks the skills or fails to honor the commitments that surgery as a profession requires. When such mistakes occur, attending physicians approach residents as wrathful and righteous judges eager to root out heresy. All those errors that are seen as blameworthy indicate that a resident is either in need of serious remediation or in need of dismissal from the training program.

One striking feature of categorizing residents' errors into the blameless and blameworthy is how easily the process may turn into a self-fulfilling prophecy. That is, a resident's good reputation exerts a protective or deviance-reducing effect while a bad one generates a destructive or deviance-amplifying effect. If a resident is considered trustworthy, monitoring by attending physicians is decreased. Therefore, deficiencies are less likely to be discovered. Conversely, if a resident is suspect, monitoring increases. Convinced that the resident's deficiencies are there for the finding, an attending physician is more likely to look for and find evidence of sloppy work. When the attending physician finds deficiencies, he or she increases surveillance, which again increases the probability of finding other mistakes. Clearly suspicion alone does not create residents who are judged unfit; after all, something creates the suspicion. Nonetheless, being suspect is for a resident a very vulnerable and demoralizing position. Not only that, being above suspicion gives a fair amount of protection, especially when mistakes need not be seen as innocent error. Given these dynamics, it is not surprising that those who fall short when evaluated (or their attorneys) often characterize the process as arbitrary and capricious.

This sense of unfairness is symbolized for residents by what I called quasi-normative errors. These are breaches of the attending physician's personal preferences, which are read as if they were absolute, universal rules. Residents who make such mistakes often find themselves locked into personality conflicts with attending physicians. Invariably, when these conflicts occur, residents are losers. There are two problems here. First, the seriousness with which these breaches of personal preference are punished undermines the seriousness of the more universal norms attending physicians seek to enforce when they react to normative error. The confusion introduced by treating personal preferences as if they were universal rules allows residents to confuse their profound and trivial lapses and to excuse too easily the serious ones. Second, this confusion is only multiplied when the quasi-normative errors of residents are simply thought of as the personal style or signature of the attending surgeon. To be sanctioned severely on one service for what is acceptable practice on another only reinforces the sense that the coding of mistakes and error is arbitrary and capricious.

Errors in Ethics Consultation

What is and is not an error, how errors occur, who is culpable, and what needs to be done to prevent their occurrence are never simply matters of defining ever more rigorously and objectively a discrete empirical event—something capable of being captured by a very sophisticated outcome measure. Rather, culpable error and its control are a matter of occupational morals, of situations defined this way rather than that, of administrative classifications about how causality works here, and of implicit social rules that make clear to all but the most obtuse when further questions are not welcome. The social constructedness of error matters, very fatefully in fact, for system participants. This is as true for pilots and airline passengers as it is for doctors and patients.

How then is error socially constructed in the world of ethics consultation? Or, to put the matter more pointedly, is it possible for a clinical ethicist to make a blameworthy error? Although it might seem nonsensical to claim that clinical ethicists do not and, in fact, cannot make blameworthy errors, this does seem to be the case. To avoid unnecessary debate, the bald assertion—the clinical bioethicist or the ethics committee is incapable of making a mistake—needs sharpening, qualifying, and clarifying. It is, possible—even likely—that for any given case the individual clinical ethicist or committee may feel that things could have been handled more smoothly, that critical opportunities were missed, or that a better outcome could have been obtained. But an ad hoc, individual sense of regret is not the same thing as an acknowledgment of error, a concrete identification of a specific mistake, and a precise mode of redress to avoid that mistake in the future. The individual clinical ethicist or ethics committee cannot make a mistake, because the structural and cognitive features that make for a shared, collective understanding of mistake are absent. The features that allow for public identification of mistakes in other occupational segments simply do not exist in the world of clinical bioethics. To those who might argue that a public, collective understanding of mistakes and errors is nothing more than a sociological rendering of these events, I would agree. And I would add that, without such a collective or sociological version of mistake and error, the community lacks the resources necessary to assess performance, redress blameworthy mistakes, and exercise the self-regulatory functions said to distinguish the professions from other occupations.

Of those missing structural and cognitive features necessary for a community's possession of an understanding of mistake and error and the capacity to act on that collective understanding when necessary—and here it is important to remember that both forgiveness and negative sanctions are actions—three are most critical. First, without any form of systematic review of problematic cases, there is no public forum in which to develop collective understanding of what counts as adequate or inadequate case management.

As Light points out, psychiatry has suicide review, which allows the community to develop standards, pinpoint errors, assess blame, forgive mistakes, and define the limits of individual clinical responsibility. Surgical morbidity and mortality conferences accomplish much of the same work in surgical departments. In these meetings, attending surgeons model and residents learn the standards of professional responsibility, the rhetoric for acceptable accounts of errors, and the boundary between acceptable and unacceptable behavior. One striking similarity between suicide review among psychiatrists and mortality and morbidity conferences among surgeons is that both meetings reassert professional claims to competence at just that moment when events most mock such claims, reassert professional standards when outcomes suggest that they have been breached, and reestablish commitment to professional norms of behavior when they seem to be most in doubt. Whatever other tasks these meetings accomplish, they are a public reaffirmation of what does and what does not count as acceptable practice and of how seriously this professional community takes those standards.

So far as I know, neither ethics consultants nor ethics committees conduct regular case reviews. There are any number of reasons for this. First, there is no outcome from ethics consultation comparable to suicide in psychiatry or mortality and morbidity in surgery. In some sense, psychiatric services are organized to prevent suicide and surgical services to avoid mortality and morbidity. When such events occur, as they inevitably will, an accounting is necessary lest it seem that the professional community is tolerant of such outcomes. But, in ethics consultation, this is not the case. There is no outcome that so challenges the professional conscience of the community that it triggers the demand for a collective, public accounting. As a consequence, there are no occupational rituals that serve to articulate, make explicit, and reinforce professional standards.[16] Without such rituals, there is no public space for an understanding of what causes a mistake or error to develop.

The absence of such occupational rituals may itself index nothing so much as how different action within the occupational community of bioethicists is from action within the community of psychiatrists and surgeons. Suicide review in psychiatry and mortality and morbidity conferences in surgery both move forward under a convenient sociological fiction—namely, outcomes are interpreted, until proven differently, as if they were determined exclusively by the actions of psychiatrist and surgeon. Certainly, the review of bioethics consultation can never proceed under this fiction. In fact, if this were true, it is not immediately clear how the consultation could subserve the value of autonomy (assuming that autonomy is one value that the consultants have an interest in preserving). Indeed, it is not even clear how fateful consultation should be in decision making. In good consultations do those whom one has consulted follow recommendations? In good consultations are recommendations given in the alternative (a set of options) with likely costs and benefits attached? Or in good consultations are no recommendations given at all? Rather, instead of concrete suggestions, are the parties to the consultation empowered to frame and assess the options themselves? So, without a clear idea of what role the consultation is supposed to play in unfolding action, it is very difficult to say that a mistake was made in consultation. Beyond that, whatever is ultimately decided in the case is not decided by the bioethicist. Typically to make a mistake or error, one must exercise some exclusive decision-making authority. Bioethicists rarely do this qua bioethicists. As a rule, it is hard to assess which streams of their clinical talk in a case are mistaken and which are correct, if only because it is so hard to connect those streams of talk to actions taken and, ultimately, to outcomes.

Finally, there is one last reason that inhibits regular case review in bioethics consultation. Both the psychiatry departments that conduct suicide review conferences and the surgery departments that hold mortality and morbidity conferences are densely peopled. From these conferences, there are impersonal lessons that can be communicated to a broader collegium. This is much less so for those units responsible for bioethics consultation. Most commonly, ethics consultation is managed through a committee. Alternatively, a hospital may have a few individuals who provide consultation services. When committees provide consultation services, it is always the case that members have other, more primary clinical responsibilities. Committee work is an additional service provided to the institution for a wide, if unspecified, range of motives. When individuals provide consulting services, it is also rarely the case that ethics consultations are their primary clinical responsibility. Under these conditions, a regular review of performance is inhibited for two reasons. First, however valuable such a review is, whatever lessons are learned from it, close case review is often stressful, time-consuming, and interpersonally difficult. Because committees need to enlist volunteers and then to motivate their continued involvement, regular case reviews with a focus on what was done wrong may seem to volunteers an undue burden, a heavy price to provide what is often a thankless, extra administrative duty. Additionally, with the ethics committee and also where a few individuals provide consultation services, there is no audience to inform beyond those who already know the details of the case for a review. In short, the community of professionals involved in ethics consultation is very rarely dense enough to support the kind of public review of outcomes found in suicide review and mortality and morbidity conferences. In such small communities of workers, it would be most difficult not to personalize criticism and to focus on impersonal lessons learned.

But even if there were formal case reviews in bioethics to dissect mistakes and to delineate measures to prevent their reoccurrence, it seems highly unlikely that these sessions would be of much value. First, there is too little consensus on what the goals of ethics consultation are. Part of what makes suicide review or mortality and morbidity conference important is that suicide and mortality and morbidity are just those events that psychiatric treatment or surgery are instituted to prevent. The comparable event for ethics consultation, the one that signals that consultation itself has been error ridden, is hard to specify. There has been an explosive growth in ethics committees and individual ethics consultants in the last decade. This growth has been fueled, in part, by the requirement of the Joint Commission on Accreditation of Healthcare Organizations (JCAHO) that institutions need to have in place a mechanism to resolve the ethical dilemmas arising in the course of care. What the JCAHO is silent about is how these mechanisms are to be organized, how they are to operate, and how institutions are to assess the efficiency of these mechanisms.

This silence presents many difficulties to anyone who wishes to assess whether ethics consultation, however it is organized, properly serves the goals it is intended to serve. The JCAHO's standard suggests that all mechanisms and all resolutions are equally acceptable. This plainly cannot be the case. An ethical dispute can be resolved by the patient's death, by a physician overriding the patient's or family's wish, or by a physician simply acceding to the patient's or family's wishes even if these wishes are morally problematic and beyond the bounds of community standards. Some of these resolutions are clearly preferable to others from the point of view of norms, social process, or both. But, ultimately, in order to assess whether mistakes or errors occurred in an ethics consultation, we would need a more certain sense of how ethics consultations are to resolve ethical conflict. Is the purpose of consultation to provide a forum for protecting the patient's autonomy? Or is ethics consultation a procedure to ensure that some specific overarching cultural values are respected? Or is ethics consultation a process designed to avoid litigation and adverse public relations for hospitals? Without a consensus on questions such as these, the judgment of an action as reasonable and responsible or fatally flawed in conception and execution is difficult, if not impossible, to make.

Knowing the goal of ethics consultation is a necessary but not a sufficient condition for determining if a mistake or error has been made in any particular case consultation. What is also needed, and in this case missing, are some data that suggest that one way of doing consultation provides better outcomes than some other way. Here our knowledge of consultation is flawed on two counts. First, at a theoretical level, there are multiple approaches to doing consultations. Consultants approach their tasks from a variety of paradigms. There are bioethics consultants deeply committed to a principlist, a narrative, a phenomenological, a dialogical, or a virtue-based approach to their work. But this in itself is not a flaw. After all, multiple paradigms exist in psychiatry where the arguments among those who favor behavioral, cognitive, pharmacological, psychodynamic, or family-system approaches to various problems are ceaseless and no less passionate on that account. Likewise, in surgery, there is no lack of debate on the proper approach to specific illnesses or procedures. What these fields possess that bioethics lacks is agreement on outcome measures and controlled clinical trials that compare different approaches. This is the second failing of bioethics consultation that makes errors and mistakes hard to gauge. Put most simply, there are no data that suggest that any one approach creates different results than another. We do not know what difference the various theoretical operating paradigms make. Beyond that, we do not know what difference the variety of ways these paradigms are implemented makes. Does it make a difference in outcomes whether consultation is by committee or by individuals? Does it matter whether patients and their families are part of the process? Does in matter whether consultants have any specific set of professionally trained competencies? Without this sort of data, it is simply impossible to say that one approach was a mistake or that errors were made.

Conclusion

In reviewing the sociology of error and then applying that sociology to bioethics consultation to conclude that consultants cannot make mistakes, I have not meant to imply that consultants are not conscientious individuals who do trying and much-needed work under difficult circumstances in often thankless environments. For it is plainly the case that ethics consultation provides a necessary corrective to many of the least praiseworthy features of modern medical care. It is equally clear that ethics consultants are dedicated, committed, and conscientious workers. Their own writings reveal that they are also self-reflective about the practice of their craft and very far from uncritical about their performance.

What I have tried to do in this essay is not look so much at individual case performance but rather provide a framework for understanding what is necessary in the occupational community of ethics consultants for a collective understanding of mistake and error to emerge—of what work is necessary to move beyond an ad hoc assessment of individual consultations. This framework includes three elements: regular case review, agreement on outcomes and a means for assessing them, and systematic data that compare different approaches to ethics consultation. It is most understandable that, in an emerging and often contested domain of professional practice, these elements have not yet developed. But, if ethics consultation is to continue in its institutionalization in healthcare organizations, these three elements demand the attention of the community of practitioners.

Notes

1. C. Perrow, *Normal Error: Living with High-Risk Technologies* (New York: Basic Books, 1985).
2. Ibid., 5.
3. D. Vaughan, *The Challenger Launch Decision: Risky Technology, Culture and Deviance at NASA* (Chicago: University of Chicago Press, 1996).
4. D. Matza, *Delinquency and Drift* (New York: John Wiley, 1964), 56.
5. J. Bensman and I. Gerver, "Crime and Punishment in the Factory: The Function of Deviance in Maintaining a Social System," *American Sociological Review* 28 (1963): 588–99.
6. D. Roy, "Quota Restriction and Goldbricking in a Machine Shop," *American Journal of Sociology* 57 (1952): 427–42; D. Roy, "Banana Time: Job Satisfaction and Informal Interaction," *Human Organization* 18 (1960): 156–68.
7. M. Lipsky, *Street-Level Bureaucracy* (New York: Russell-Sage, 1980).
8. M. Dalton, *Men Who Manage* (New York: John Wiley, 1959).
9. E. C. Hughes, "Mistakes at Work," in *The Sociological Eye: Selected Papers on Work, Self, and Society* (Chicago: Aldine-Atherton, 1951, 1971), 316–25.
10. P. Atkinson, "Training for Uncertainty," *Social Science & Medicine* 19 (1984): 949–56.
11. M. Paget, *The Unity of Mistakes: The Phenomenological Interpretation of Medical Work* (Philadelphia: Temple University Press, 1988).
12. C. West, *Routine Complications: Troubles with Talk between Doctors and Patients* (Bloomington, Ind.: Indiana University Press, 1984).

13. D. Light, "Psychiatry and Suicide: The Management of a Mistake," *American Sociological Review* 77 (1972): 821–38.

14. Ibid., 835.

15. C. L. Bosk, *Forgive and Remember: Managing Medical Failure* (Chicago: University of Chicago Press, 1979).

16. Ibid.

FIVE

Bureaucracies of Mass Deception

INSTITUTIONAL REVIEW BOARDS AND THE ETHICS
OF ETHNOGRAPHIC RESEARCH

Charles L. Bosk and Raymond G. De Vries

One score and seven years ago, the National Commission for the Protection of Human Subjects of Biomedical and Behavioral Research met in February to identify the ethical principles that would serve as guidelines for the protection of human subjects of biomedical and behavioral research. The discussions from those meetings culminated in the *Belmont Report*. In the summer of 2003, The Social and Behavioral Sciences Working Group on Human Research Protections convened a conference at, fittingly enough, the Belmont Conference Center. The title of the conference was *IRB [Institutional Review Board] Best Practices in the Review of Social and Behavioral Research*; the working group invited a collection of persons—with "considerable expertise in human research protections and the review of social and behavioral science protocols"—to join them at the Belmont Center. Topics for the various sessions of the conference included "IRBs that Work"; "Back to the Basics for Social and Behavioral Research," that is, what is and what is not research,

Chapter 5 was originally published as Charles L. Bosk and Raymond G. De Vries, "Bureaucracies of Mass Deception: IRBs and the Ethics of Ethnographic Research," in *Being Here and Being There: Fieldwork Encounters and Ethnographic Discoveries*, ed. Elijah Anderson, Scott N. Brooks, Raymond Gunn, and Nikki Jones. *The Annals of the American Academy of Political and Social Science* 595, no.l (Sept. 2004) Sage Publications, 249–63.

the meaning of generalizable knowledge to subjects, the concept of the human subject; "Challenging Protocols—Methods of Inquiry"; "Challenging Protocols—Contexts and Populations"; "Barriers in Reviewing Protocols"; "Best Practices in the Consideration of Consent, Disclosure, and Deception"; and "Research Risk and Best Practices in the Determination of Exempt and Expedited Review." The Office of Behavioral and Social Science Research of the National Institutes of Health provided support for the conference.

It is difficult to fully assess how successful the participants were in identifying "best practices."[1] Since the conference itself was held a mere six months before we began writing this article, it is too soon to say how effectively the results of the conference will be disseminated or, for that matter, to whom. If the goals of the conference were to identify a set of best practices, to operationalize those practices in a set of procedures, and to distribute those procedures as a set of guidelines to those in academic or commercial organizations with responsibility for administration and compliance with federal regulations, then there is no reason to expect anything less than a successful outcome. Working groups experienced in the production of such documents can produce guidelines on most anything. Administrators charged with translating vague principles into coherent procedures often find such documents a great comfort. At the very least, guidelines stored in a binder and filed on a shelf provide grounds for arguing later about whether institutions discharged responsibilities properly.[2] However, if the working group hoped that conference participants would help produce a document that quells the considerable resentment that the bureaucratic regulation of research has created among social scientists, then they are likely to be severely disappointed, no matter how sensible, adequate, and nonintrusive the recommendations are. In fact, for those whose behaviorthe guidelines seek to regulate, the mere existence of one more document trying to get right the vexing question of how to assure the proper ethical conduct of qualitative researchers through organizational oversight is a symbol and symptom of a deep misunderstanding of the realities of ethnographic research and an even deeper misapprehension about how conduct is effectively regulated. In the current environment, one more working group's recommendations are more likely to fuel rather than to extinguish the flames of discontent. The burden of this article is to illustrate why this is so.

Some of the reasons for this are structural. First, social and behavioral research encompasses a vast amount of ground to cover with a single set of regulations. Just how vast this ground is becomes clear when we look at the membership of the Social and Behavioral Sciences Working Group on Human Research Protections, the well-intended conveners of the second Belmont Conference on the ethical conduct of research. The working group had representatives from demography, education, family and community medicine, sociology, and psychology.[3] The working group also includes representatives from numerous federal agencies who fund or conduct social and behavioral science research: the National Institutes of Health, the Federal Bureau of Prisons, the Department of Education, the National Science Foundation, and the Agency for International Development. The executive officers of the American Sociological Association and the American Education Research Association are also members of the working group. Those charged with applying regulations are also represented in the working group composition—there is an associate dean for research, a director of ethics education, and a director of a Native American research and training center.

Even with this extensive disciplinary and organizational coverage, qualitative research is underrepresented in the membership of the working group. One member of the working group, who attended the conference, mentions in his or her biographical sketch participating in projects using a wide range of methodologies from clinical trials to ethnographic research but then claims a special expertise in "the distribution and use of public-use data files," an important topic to be sure but not one that is reassuring to those who desire to see the special problems that research regulations present to ethnographers fully understood, adequately described, and realistically addressed. In all fairness, the list of attendees at the conference supplemented the expertise of the working group—qualitative researchers from sociology, anthropology, and political science participated in the conference. But the influence of these participants in the documents prepared by the working group remains to be seen. This structural flaw in representation is a generic one for tasks where a consensus that satisfies a vast array of interest groups needs to be reached, but to promote effective deliberation, the size of the working group must be limited. Still, to assemble a working group without a symbolic representative of those practitioners within the social sciences—ethnographers, who have grumbled and groused the loudest about the hindrances that the current regulatory structure imposes—seems to be a grave tactical error. After all, conversion and co-optation are, as ethnographers of deviance and social control have demonstrated, two very effective strategies for neutralizing problem populations.[4] The voices of social scientists who have complaints about IRBs and their operation deserve a fuller hearing.

If the problem of representation is a generic structural problem, the title of the conference reflects a second structural problem, quite specific to social and behavioral science research of the qualitative kind.[5] To title the conference *IRB Best Practices* is to link the regulation of social science research with the current regulatory regimes of clinical medicine, supported by rationales drawn from evidence-based medicine. Conferences or research aimed at identifying best practices have become a staple of the modern world of medical practice, especially in those domains that attempt to link clinical practice to findings supported by "outcomes research." The language of best practices is part of the Quality Improvement (QI) or Total Quality Improvement (TQI) movement in medicine. The aspirational goals of this movement are entirely laudable; it seeks to adapt some of the management practices from other industries into medicine to create a more efficient, effective, and safer system for health care delivery. The title of the conference, then, reinforces the link between the rules that regulate biomedical research and the rules that regulate social and behavioral science research. For many social scientists, this linkage is precisely the problem.

IRBs can develop best practices for routine review and approval of qualitative research proposals; however, many in the social science community feel that those best practices will never be good practices so long as research is modeled on the standard clinical trial. Even if the conference conveners intended to move away from the clinical model, the banner under which the conference was convened belies their intention. In the standard research proposal, a hypothesis or set of hypotheses about the effect of intervention x on condition y is being tested. The researcher generally has a clearly bounded relationship with the research subject. The procedures involved, their risks and benefits, and the alternatives can usually be described in some detail.[6] Roles, rules, and procedures are clear and time limited. Subjects can be fully informed, a goal that is realized more in the breach than in the fact.[7] For some types of social science research—the laboratory experiment, the fixed-item survey, the longitudinal panel study—the relationship of researcher and subject closely tracks the biomedical model that informs IRB procedures: a highly structured, objective relationship.[8]

But ethnographic research fits this model poorly. For ethnographers, the primary data-gathering tool consists of the relationships that we forge with those whose lifeworld we are trying to understand. Few of us start with specific hypotheses that we will later test in any systematic way. Furthermore, to the degree that we can restate our disciplinary curiosity as a set of testable propositions, these hypotheses are likely to be trivial. We cannot state our procedures any more formally than we will hang around here in this particular neighborhood and try to figure out what is going on among these people. We want to know how they make sense of their world, how they navigate in it, and how understanding their world helps us better understand our own. Neighborhoods vary: this store that serves as front for the crack dealers (Bourgois 1995); these clubs where the blues musicians congregate (Grazian 2003); this neonatal intensive-care unit (Anspach 1993; Heimer and Stauffen 1998); these neighborhoods where people sell their kidneys (Cohen 1999); these laboratories where biologists seek to unravel the mystery of peptides (Latour and Woolgar 1986). Neighborhoods change but methods are remarkably constant—really, they have not changed much for sociologists since Whyte (1942) or for anthropologists since Malinowski (1922).[9] We observe, we may tape-record, we may videotape, we all take notes, and we code those notes according to our own various schemas—some of us use computers to sort data, and some of us still cut and paste and shuffle file cards.[10] We do not know in advance what questions we will ask or, for that matter, where we will draw a curtain and choose not to inquire—or decide not to report.

We cannot inform our subjects of the risks and benefits of cooperating with us for a number of reasons. First, the risks and benefits for subjects are not so different from those of normal interaction with a stranger who will become a close acquaintance, an everyday feature of a lifeworld, and then disappear, after observing intimate moments, exploring deep feelings, and asking embarrassing questions. There is the risk inherent in any fleeting human relationship—the risk of bruised feelings that come from being used, the loss when a fixture in a social world disappears, or the hurt of realizing that however differently it felt in the moment, one was used as a means to an end.[11] This risk is magnified by a certain unavoidable deception in every ethnographic investigation, a certain pretense that comes from trying to have both researcher and informant forget that what is going on is not a normal, natural exchange but research—not just everyday life as it naturally occurs but work, a job, a project—"No really, I'm interested in what you have to say, think, feel, and believe for more than my own narrow instrumental academic purposes." To some degree, we cannot specify risks because we do not know what we will find, what interpretive frameworks we will develop for reporting what we do observe, and how the world around us will change to make those findings seem more or less significant.[12] Finally, we cannot define risk because few of us believe that being an ethnographic informant is a risky business. We believe this despite considerable anthropological and sociological evidence to the contrary.

IRBs also review proposals to make sure that the confidentiality and anonymity of study subjects is adequately safeguarded. In general, this last element is relatively easy to promise. However, some situations are highly problematic. For those of us who work with highly literate populations, confidentiality and anonymity are much easier to promise than to assure. We can do nothing to prohibit a sufficiently determined reader from trying to decode the text, to stop a figure in an ethnographic narrative from identifying himself or herself, or to prevent an institution from coming forward and saying, "We are 'made-up-ville'" (Bosk 2000).[13] Typically, such decodings are harmless but not necessarily. If read as romans à clef, ethnographic works among hospital workers can make tense and fractious workplaces even tenser and more fractious for the workers within them, who now know what they previously only suspected, who see on the printed page what was once said only behind closed doors.

In anthropology, regimes already in place have used the "thick descriptions" of ethnographic works to root out troublesome populations. This has happened despite the best efforts of anthropologists to foresee risks to subjects and to veil identities. Political climates change. What seemed a harmless remark yesterday may appear to be an insurrectionary one tomorrow. A group that no one seemed to care about can grow central when regimes shift. In addition, the requirement of subject confidentiality and anonymity, if stretched too far, does not permit ethnographic work in public domains. The workings of government, for instance, at the local, state, or federal level, would be hamstrung by an overly rigid insistence on confidentiality and anonymity. Certain forms of public controversy could not be explored as well. Because of the risks posed when confidentiality and anonymity are breached, IRBs, at least in the minds of researchers, have imposed consent requirements that themselves are out of character with the type of research being proposed. Bruner (2004) provides two different examples: (1) being asked to get written consent from illiterate peoples and (2) having colleagues refuse to answer questions about difficulties with IRBs until they were assured that the inquiry itself had been sanctioned by an IRB.[14]

So to restate the obvious, social scientists and behavioral scientists, in general, and ethnographers, in particular, are not thrilled with current federal regulations that require prospective review of research projects; they are skeptical that such review improves the ethical quality of research; and they believe that such review does nothing more than hinder the pace of research. Truth be told, medical researchers have never been much thrilled with the regulations either. They have done their public grousing and grumbling, and generally, they have figured out what it is that IRBs want to hear and figured out ways to say exactly that. Since IRB review is almost entirely prospective, there exists very little check on whether researchers in clinical domains do exactly what they say they are going to do.[15] Why have social and behavioral science researchers not done the same? Why have they not adopted a policy of weary, self-resigned compliance coupled with minor or major evasion? Or even, if they have used passive-aggressive strategies of compliance and evasion, why are there also so many public complaints and so many public calls for resistance?

Both the complaints and the calls for resistance seem peculiar on any number of counts. First, there is an inaccurate stridency to some of the complaints. Some of those who are opposed to the current regime of IRB research have complained that the regulations violate a First Amendment right to unfettered speech. This absolute interpretation of the First Amendment neglects the considerable jurisprudence that indicates that reasonable restrictions might be placed on the time, place, and manner of speech. Others have complained that journalists, especially those journalists who do investigative reporting, are not hemmed by requirements for informed consent or the need to respect confidentiality. Why should sociological researchers, they ask, be held to a higher standard? One deceptively simple answer is that perhaps we should aspire to a higher standard than the average journalist. Journalism is, after all, a commercial enterprise, many of the workers in which lack what are often thought of as the prerequisites of a professional occupation—long adult socialization in a specialized body of theoretic knowledge.[16] Journalism is not supported by public funds. Because we are not journalists, however many similarities one can identify between ethnographic research and investigative journalism, we have no reason to expect the same rules to apply.

Next, something is vaguely uncollegial and distasteful to the social scientist's objections to IRBs on two counts. First, much of the social science critique of both the research and the clinical practices of physicians centers on how poorly patients or subjects are informed of what is being done to them, why it is being done, and what alternatives exist. Freidson (1970), for one, has argued that physicians have used their technical authority as scientific experts to make normative decisions, choices that patients or research subjects ought to make for themselves in a democratic society. The early sociological writing on death and dying (Glaser and Strauss 1968) stressed how much information control by physicians robbed patients of autonomy and dignity. Emerson (1969) characterized the desperate measures that patients used to try to gain accurate information on their conditions. Davis (1960) described how physicians manipulated and feigned uncertainty to control and limit patient choices. Sociologists decried these practices of information control. To a degree, when coupled with the revelations of past ethical abuses such as those Beecher (1966) catalogued or those that revealed the suffering of vulnerable, minority populations at Tuskegee (Jones 1981), these critiques led to the recommendations of the first Belmont report (Rothman 1991) that stressed informing patients so that they could reasonably exercise decision-making capacity.[17] There is more than a whiff of hypocrisy in imposing obligations on others—in this case, physicians and medical researchers who cannot be trusted because their self-interest makes unreliable their judgments of others' best interests—while resisting those very same obligations for oneself because our work is harmless, our intentions good, and our hearts pure.

A second dimension of the uncollegial spirit of the social and behavioral reaction to IRB review is its uncharitable nature. If we were honest, we would recognize that IRBs and the regulatory and administrative regimes for research now have a fair amount of bureaucratic momentum behind them. How much good IRBs accomplish and how much harm they prevent remain open questions. How procedures might evolve so that they better meet the realities and contingencies of social and behavioral research as it is actually done in a real world of real people is certainly open. What is not open is whether a prospective review of research will exist.[18] So at the very least, we social scientists ought to recognize that the committee work that involves our colleagues on IRBs is like a lot of other committee work. It is thankless; it is done in pursuit of some communally shared objectives, even if these are poorly articulated; it is underfunded; and if it were not done by these colleagues, we might have to do it ourselves, which would mean that we would have less time to do our own research. We should all, then, be a bit more forgiving of the imperfections of the whole structure even as we remember them—all the better to correct them. If all this were not reason enough to be a bit more constructive and cooperative in our critique of IRBs, we can add one more: none of us truly objects to the goals of IRB review—we all wish subjects to be treated with respect, protected from harm, and saved from embarrassing exposure.

Therefore, we need some constructive suggestions for making the system work better, we need to educate IRB members about the nature of qualitative social science research, and we need to do a better job of educating ourselves about the regulations—if only because such education will make clear to us that the system is less onerous than we fear. We need to explore the different ways that the system can be streamlined and made more efficient. It is in this spirit that we offer the following suggestions, all of which have been floated in the vast literature on IRBs.

Encourage more and better studies of how IRBs work · Given the continued and high level of displeasure with IRBs, we would expect ethnographers to be studying the way IRBs work. When it comes to IRBs, social scientists are cobbler's children. Like the hapless waifs whose feet remain unshod while their parent makes shoes for others, social scientists complain about the many shortcomings of IRBs while using their skills to describe and analyze nearly every other sphere of human activity. Reports on the shortcomings of IRBs are rarely supported by data. A recent American Association of University Professors (2001) report is based on anecdote, a nonscientific survey of social science researchers, and testimony given to government committees; the report of the National Research Council lists only eight studies in an appendix, "Selected Studies of IRB Operations: Summary Descriptions." One might assume this small number is the result of careful selection, but as the authors of the study note, "There is little regularly available systematic information about the functioning of the U.S. human research participant protection system" (Citro, Ilgen, and Marrett 2003). We need to better understand what IRBs look like and how they work (De Vries and Forsberg 2002).

Increase social scientist participation on IRBs · In institutions with multiple subcommittees of IRBs, create a specialized IRB for vetting social science research. IRB composition has specific requirements: multiple disciplines must be represented, there must be a community representative, and there must be at least five members. There is no reason why one subcommittee cannot specialize in social science research. This will assure that research is reviewed by colleagues who have some understanding of social science methodologies.

Increase social scientists' knowledge of IRB rules · We all need greater understanding of what the rules require of us. A good deal of ethnographic research falls under the category of expedited or exempt research. We need to familiarize ourselves with these categories of research. We need to make clear to IRBs why we believe that our research falls into one category or the other. We need to be familiar with those situations where the regulations allow something other than written consent; generally, in situations of minimal risk, alternatives to written consent are permissible. We also need to know which populations are defined as vulnerable and the set of special protections afforded such populations.

From experiences as a member of study sections for the Ethical, Legal and Social Implications part of the Human Genome Project, one of us often found that researchers submitting proposals using qualitative research methods are defensive when specifying what they will do and are incomplete when discussing consent procedures. As a consequence, methods are left vaguer than they need to be, and the requirements for consent appear to be evaded rather than embraced. We understand why this happens: it is a pain (really, there is no other word for it) to try to shape a proposal for a qualitative research effort into the format required by a National Institutes of Health RO1 Grant application. But if we wish funding for our projects, it is a pain we must endure. Specifying to an IRB how we will meet the requirements of informed consent is likewise a pain, but it is one that can be borne with a bit more grace than we have managed so far. We can begin to engage the process creatively if we know the rules. The more familiar we become with those rules, the more we can work around them, find the loopholes, and yes, even amend them so that they make sense given the kinds of inquiry in which we engage.

Educate IRB members · Social scientists have complained about the "mission creep" that occurred when IRB jurisdiction expanded from biomedical research to all research involving human subjects. Whether this truly was mission creep or just a natural extension of a mandate is for others to debate and decide; however, the fact that IRBs began to review proposals with biomedical research in mind has had a number of implications for social scientists using qualitative methods. First, the personnel who serve on IRBs are, as a consequence, overwhelmingly drawn from the ranks of biomedical researchers.[19] Research protocols themselves are then reviewed in narrow terms: What was the risk/benefit ratio? How adequate was the consent form? When faced with qualitative research proposals, whatever normal operating procedures and rules for deliberation committees had evolved break down. In addition, the template of the research being proposed makes little scientific sense to committee members who have a trained incompetence when it comes to the inductive methods of qualitative research. Under these conditions, too many IRBs have members who decide that qualitative research has no scientific validity; hence, it can offer no benefit; and as a consequence, there is no risk worth contemplating for human subjects. Qualitative researchers then have reasonable proposals turned back with what seems like a set of unreasonable objections and appears to be a willful obtuseness about the nature, conduct, and purpose of the proposed research. To avoid this situation, two types of education for IRB members are required. First, IRB members need to learn to extend beyond their own disciplinary boundaries. They need not like, approve, or be advocates for qualitative research. They do need, however, to have enough education in its methods and the theories of social life that undergird them to appreciate that this is a legitimate form of inquiry. With this understanding comes the knowledge that there are better and worse ways to proceed with qualitative projects, that there are criteria of judgment that can be applied, and that reasoned decisions can be made rather than positivistic prejudices enacted. Second, IRB members, like their social science counterparts, need to be familiar with their own rules of operation. They need to know which research qualifies as minimal risk, which projects are exempt from review and which can receive expedited review, and which research projects are allowed alternatives to written consent. If IRB members are not well versed in the rules that they are charged with applying, then they will have difficulty applying those rules correctly.

Have in place a speedy appeals process · One thing that frustrates researchers, whatever methods they employ, is delays encountered when IRB approval stalls the start of projects. For qualitative researchers, this frustration is multiplied when it seems that a failure to win approval grows out of a misreading in what was involved in the research process. Resubmissions that require answering nonsensical objections are not an adequate remedy. For the requirements imposed to make a research proposal pass muster may also make that same project impossible to do. Beyond that, the delay between original submission, response to objection, and resubmission may erode whatever access to a field setting that has been negotiated. Finally, there is little confidence that the same folks who made such a seemingly arbitrary decision so recently will now act with the requisite wisdom. Institutions need to have in place appeals mechanisms that allow researchers a speedy hearing before a body of colleagues who will not be made defensive or be constrained by their prior rulings, who understand what qualitative methods entail, and who are familiar with the rules governing research with human subjects. IRBs need to remember that few researchers design projects with the intent of harming people. Researchers need to remember that IRBs have a specific job to do. An appeals process that puts the ball in a different court reminds each of them that neither of them is infallible.

Explore other ways of organizing review of social science research · The United States was a pioneer in the creation of ethics review boards, but we have much to learn from the ways other countries have responded to the need to protect the subjects of research. There are other ways to organize ethics reviews and other ways to approach review of social science research. In the Netherlands, for example, social science research is exempt from review unless it places a demonstrable physical or psychological burden on its subjects. Paying attention to the way our colleagues in other countries have approached this problem will create solutions to our dilemmas.[20]

So that is the gist of the argument. IRBs are here to stay. The review process may impose more harm than benefit, but it is hard to imagine turning back now. Social scientists are not bureaucratic incompetents or mutes. They can find ways to work within the system at the same time that they work to change it. When the requirements for approving research with minimal risk are looked at, the entire review process seems to impose fewer burdens than what we actually complain about. The system is highly imperfect. We can make it better. The system is underfunded and understaffed. Given this, a spirit of cooperation rather than belligerence seems the appropriate way to respond to our colleagues who have either volunteered or had their arms twisted to perform this onerous task.

All that said, we cannot help but feel that one more thing is worth saying. We do not think that the system of prospective review that we have adopted does much to protect subjects from harm or guarantee ethical conduct from researchers. The ethical problems that we meet in the field are so complex and the situations are so fraught with the moral and existential dilemmas of leading a life that consent does little to assure our subjects or ourselves, for that matter, that we will do the right thing when the situation presents itself. What should the sociologist studying faith healing in suburban New Jersey do when parents refuse to take a sick child to the physician? What does the sociologist studying an intensive-care unit say when a doctor, nurse, or family member contemplating treatment withdrawal asks what he or she should do? What does the anthropologist studying the drug-addicted homeless do when an informant, copping some heroin, is a few dollars short and asks for a loan? In his book *The Secret Army: The IRA, 1916–1974*, J. Bowyer Bell (1970) includes a series of photographs depicting a bomb attack.[21] Four plates detail the loading of the bomb into the car, the moments before the explosion, the explosion itself, and the damage done. It turns out that these photographs were not taken by Bowyer Bell, but one can easily imagine that the qualitative researcher studying a group like the IRA, or a teen gang, or professional gamblers, or sex workers would come upon such scenes. In scenes when the last item in the sequence is "the damage done," it is certainly reasonable to ask what are the obligations of the researcher to his or her informants, as well as to third parties. Resolving this sort of ethical dilemma is not the sort of thing that is amenable to prospective review, to an abstract calculation of risks and benefits, and to consent. The problem with IRBs for qualitative research is that they are such a distraction from the real difficulties that we face and from the real ethical dilemmas that confront us that we may not recognize and discuss the serious and elemental because we are so busy with the procedural and bureaucratic.

References

Alther, Lisa. 1976. *Kinflicks*. New York: Knopf.

American Association of University Professors. 2001. Protecting human beings: Institutional review boards and social science research. *Academe* 87 (3): 55–67. Also available at http://www.aaup.org/statements/ Redbook/repirb.htm.

Anspach, Renee. 1993. *Deciding who lives: Fateful choices in the intensive-care nursery.* Berkeley: University of California Press.

Beecher, Henry K. 1966. Ethics and clinical research. *New England Journal of Medicine* 74:1354–60.

Bell, J. Bowyer. 1970. *The secret army: The IRA, 1916–1970.* London: Blond.

Bosk, Charles L. 2000. Irony, ethnography, and informed consent. In *Bioethics in social context*, edited by Barry C. Hoffmaster, 199–220. Philadelphia: Temple University Press.

Bourgois, Phillippe. 1995. *In search of respect: Selling crack in El Barrio.* New York: Cambridge University Press.

Bruner, Edward. 2004. Ethnographic practice and human subjects review. *Anthropology Newsletter*, January.

Citro, C. F., D. R. Ilgen, and C. B. Marrett, eds. 2003. *Protecting participants and facilitating social and behavioral sciences research.* Washington, DC: National Academies Press.

Cohen, Lawrence. 1999. Where it hurts: Indian material for an ethics of organ trans-plantation. *Daedalus* 128 (4): 135–66.

Davis, Fred. 1960. Uncertainty in medical diagnosis: Clinical and functional. *American Journal of Sociology* 66:41–47.

De Vries, Raymond. Forthcoming. How can we help? From "sociology in" to "sociology of" bioethics. *Journal of Law, Medicine and Ethics.*

De Vries, Raymond, and Carl Forsberg. 2002. What do IRBs look like? What kind of support do they receive? *Accountability in Research* 9:199–216.

Emerson, Joan. 1969. Negotiating the serious import of humor. *Sociometry* 32:169–81.

Freidson, Eliot. 1970. *The profession of medicine: A study in the sociology of applied knowledge.* New York: Harper and Row.

———. 1975. *Doctoring together.* New York: Elsevier.

Glaser, Barney, and Anselm Strauss. 1968. *Time for dying.* Chicago: Aldine.

Goldfarb, Jeffrey. 1982. *On cultural freedom: An exploration of public life in Poland and America.* Chicago: University of Chicago Press.

Grazian, David. 2003. *Blue Chicago: The search for authenticity in Chicago blues clubs.* Chicago: University of Chicago Press.

Heimer, Carole, and Lisa Stauffen. 1998. *For the sake of the children: The social organization of responsibility in the hospital and the home.* Chicago: University of Chicago Press.

Jones, James. 1981. *Bad blood: The Tuskegee syphilis experiment.* New York: Free Press.

Latour, Bruno, and Steve Woolgar. 1986. *Laboratory life: The construction of scientific facts.* Princeton, NJ: Princeton University Press.

Malinowski, Bruno. 1922. *Argonauts of the Western Pacific.* London: Routledge.

Parsons, Talcott. 1951. *The social system.* New York: Free Press.

Petryna, Adriana. Forthcoming. The human subjects research industry. In *Global pharmaceuticals: Ethics, markets, practices,* edited by Adriana Petryna, Andrew Lakoff, and Arthur Kleinman.

Rothman, David. 1991. *Strangers at the bedside: A history of how law and bioethics transformed medical decision-making.* New York: Basic Books.

Snook, Scott. 2000. *Friendly fire: The accidental shootdown of U.S. Blackhawks over Northern Iraq.* Princeton, NJ: Princeton University Press.

Whyte, William F. 1942. *Street corner society.* Chicago: University of Chicago Press.

Notes

1. One of us (De Vries) was present at the conference. Attendees generated useful and long lists of (1) the problems of reviewing the research proposals of social and behavioral scientists and (2) the solutions to those problems; staff members of the working group are in the process of refining these lists.

2. A wise law school faculty member once told one of us (Bosk) that contracts do not regulate working relationships among parties. When there is an adequate working relationship, there is no need for a contract—the parties

can work out differences on the hoof as it were. In fact, that ability to make adjustments and move on is as good an operational definition of a working relationship as one might ever hope to find. Contracts set the ground rules for the dispute when working relationships fall apart. Guidelines are a bit the same; it is only when disaster fails to be averted that one needs to check if guidelines were followed. One consequence of this is, as Snook (2000) points out, that there is a great deal of organizational drift in everyday practice as the need for practical contingencies gets dislodged from formal organizational rules.

3. Anthropology, political science, social work, and nursing are nowhere to be found in the individual disciplines of the working-group members or among the professional associations with representatives on the working group. A note from the editors in the January 2004 issue of *Anthropology News* informs readers that "work on a position paper defining ethnographic practice with reference to IRB [institutional review board] guidelines has been begun by the AAA [American Anthropological Association]" (p. 10).

4. There are two other groups that went unrepresented. Here, the lack of representation is likely to go unnoticed, but it is not unimportant on that account. First, there were no representatives from the increasing number of organizations that provide institutional review board (IRB) review of protocols for a fee. Second, there were no representatives of commercial research organizations, a fast-growing organizational segment within the research marketplace that is responsible for a good deal of social and behavioral research in the clinical/medical domain (e.g., research on compliance with medication regimes; Petryna, forthcoming).

5. Identifying this problem, as one that is specific to "social and behavioral research of a qualitative kind," points to another larger, definitional problem, hiding behind the problem of representation. There are multiple kinds of qualitative techniques. Calling interview studies ethnographies, or identifying focus groups as a technique for providing a "thick description," does little to solve the confusions induced when trying to write rules that assure that firsthand observational research conducted in settings where behavior naturally occurs—research that cannot be done effectively without rapport, trust, assent, and consent of subjects—is "ethical."

6. Here, one might need to exercise caution. Even with the medical model, the identification of risk to both research subjects and IRB members often depends on the thoroughness of the investigator, the completeness of the literature review, and the willingness of the researcher to provide what Weber called, in a far different context, "inconvenient facts." A healthy subject died in an asthma trial at Johns Hopkins when researchers failed to discover for themselves or failed to inform the IRB and, surely, as a consequence, failed to inform a volunteer in a clinical trial that a pulmonary antagonist intended to induce asthma so that the efficacy of a new therapeutic agent could be tested had caused death in animal trials. Even in the most straightforward and mechanical of research designs, the adequacy of regulations rests on what Parsons (1951) called the "institutionalized integrity" of the profession—its willingness to face inconvenient facts. To state the same

point a slightly different way, Freidson (1970, 1975) long recognized that the monitoring, surveillance, and social control of those who possess highly specialized, abstract, esoteric, theoretic knowledge depends on the cooperation of those with that knowledge. To Plato's old question, "Quis custos custodes?" (Who governs the governors?), the answer appears to be the *custodes* themselves.

7. Since the implementation of IRBs, there has been a body of evaluative research that documents the gap between the goals of the regulatory schema and their fulfillment. This research documents that consent forms are difficult to parse (the standard aimed for is that of the average eighth-grade reader), that subjects fail to understand the nature of research (double-blind nature of clinical trials is particularly problematic), and that subjects conflate the roles of researcher and clinician, as well as the nature of research and therapy. So when we say that ethnography poses special problems for IRBs that clinical research does not, we are not comparing a system that works perfectly in one domain but fails to fit another.

8. Even here, the relationship is not perfect. For example, forced-compliance studies like the Asch or Milgram experiments—and here we are leaving aside all the other ethical questions that surround these experiments, as well as the enormous lore that mis-describes them—could hardly have been practiced without deception. This, we suppose, means they are great fodder for the conference session on "Best Practices: Consent, Deception, and Disclosure." For a hilarious send-up of what it must have been like to be a subject in the Asch experiments, see the description in the novel *Kinflicks* (Alther 1976). In fact, the general requirement of informed consent—disclosure of the purpose of the study—poses problems at many levels for social scientists of all stripes. A great deal hinges on how complete the disclosure needs to be to satisfy the requirements of informed consent.

9. We could have invoked Park and Boas. Origins are tricky things. We cannot speak at all authoritatively about anthropology. We are not historians of social science. But as sociological researchers using qualitative methods, self-consciousness about what is happening here seems to us to begin with Whyte's second edition of *Street Corner Society,* published in 1955.

10. Our methods have not changed, but in both sociology and anthropology, there is a considerable amount of self-reflexiveness that has developed relatively recently about those methods. There is rather more of this in anthropology than in sociology, but in both fields, there is a rather thorough chewing over of such questions as what does it mean to represent "the other," whose voice does the ethnographer authentically represent, and whose interests do ethnographic representations represent.

11. This is phrased to deliberately echo the violation of Kant's categorical imperative. Careful readers will notice that the word *solely* has been omitted; this surely makes an ethical difference.

12. Two examples serve to illustrate this point. One is drawn from reality; one is hypothetical. Jeffrey Goldfarb's (1982) work on art and theater in Poland obtained a salience when the Solidarity movement became politically active and visible that the work did not have when he designed his study. Second,

imagine the ethnographer studying the integration of the Arab American community in the United States and its continuing ties to countries of origin before 9/11 and after 9/11.

13. All of these forms of decoding have consequences. A reader who decodes a text, incorrectly or correctly, may cause others to give pause before consenting to observational studies. An individual who, or an institution that, comes forward vitiates the promises that the researcher made to all the others in the study who have not chosen to come forward.

14. This second example highlights the difficulty of what is research and what is not. We wish to know if a group of colleagues share a problem with us because we wish to know if we are dealing with a "private trouble" or a "public issue." At what point does my inquiry shift from purely personal curiosity to a formally organized search for generalized knowledge? Or, to put it another way, are we, as Bruner fears, reaching a point where "we will not be able to have conversations about research with our colleagues without IRB approval"?

15. A new bureaucratic level of scrutiny, the data safety monitoring board (DSMB), has been created to make sure that research is as safe as promised; how well these boards will work in practice remains to be seen. Once again, like all such reporting schemes, the efficacy of DSMBs depends on the institutionalized integrity of researchers both recognizing and reporting adverse events.

16. Compare the importance of graduate training to on-the-job training in sociology or journalism. It is hard to imagine sociologists without Ph.D.s holding down positions at major research universities. On the other hand, journalists need not have attended journalism school or have advanced degrees to obtain positions of respectability. Of course, lines that are drawn sharply can be just as easily blurred. Robert Park, one of sociology's first advocates for the primary observation of social life in natural settings, came to sociology from journalism. But he did attend and receive a doctorate from a German university.

17. In a recent online article in *Spiked*, Richard Shweder has argued that the historical evidence does not support the accepted narrative of Tuskegee as racist, deceptive, and unethical research. Shweder offers a counternarrative that attempts to argue that Tuskegee was not so bad as to justify the regulatory regimes justified in its name. Whatever the merits of Shweder's argument, it is hard not to feel that the point of the article is not to correct the historical record but rather to undermine the justifications for the federal oversight of research with human subjects (available at http://www .spiked-online.com/articles/0000000CA34A.htm/).

18. We put up with quite a bit of bureaucratic nonsense as academics. We sit on strategic planning committees whose documents are often ignored or risible—we will strive for intellectual excellence and equip our students with the skills they need to excel in the world of the twenty-first century and with the skills necessary for life long learning. We participate in external and internal departmental reviews. We sit and try to figure out what the general requirement in liberal arts education means and how it can best

be accomplished. We go to faculty meetings and discuss the same inanities in the same inane way month after month, year after year. We may feel the occasional moment of self-pity about all this; we may joke about it. But, at some level, we all recognize that these sorts of meetings only seem pointless; we recognize that they are a way of discussing what kind of community we have been, we are, and we hope to be. The discussion of research ethics in IRBs is the same kind of community-making discussion, but curiously, we social scientists have some trouble recognizing this even as we debate among ourselves how much and which Durkheim our students ought to read.

19. So much was this the case that when Bosk came to Penn and became a member of the IRB there, he was designated an outside community member. This seemed strange not only to Bosk but to a federal regulator, although it took two years for Bosk to be redefined as a token for disciplinary breadth. In their recent survey of IRBs, De Vries and Forsberg (2002) found that IRBs are dominated by those working in medical occupations.

20. De Vries (forthcoming) contrasts the requirements for membership on IRBs in the Netherlands and in the United States, observing how the regulations in the United States are based on *identity*, while those in the Netherlands are based on *expertise*.

21. We would like to thank Michael Walzer for pointing us to this volume.

2

THE ETHICS OF ETHNOGRAPHY

GENETIC COUNSELORS REVISITED

SIX

Invitation to Ethnography

What should couples with Huntington's chorea do about childbearing? What do genetic counselors advise them to do? Are there genetic grounds for compelling a couple to have a so-called therapeutic abortion? How are birth defects explained to parents who bear children with these defects? In *All God's Mistakes*, I shall report on how these problems were managed in one workgroup: a genetic counseling team in an elite urban medical center. These observations are the empirical basis for a sociological discussion of problems in applying new technologies of prenatal monitoring and diagnosis. They serve as well as a springboard for considering the rights and responsibilities, duties and obligations embedded in role relationships.

I collected the primary data during two intensive periods of participant observation among a team of genetic counselors who invited me to join them because they were aware that the services they offered patients were bound to involve questions of a social sort.[1] These services included counseling couples who either already had, or were believed to be at risk for having, a genetically defective offspring, as well as diagnostic testing. At the time of observation, no treatments for defects discovered *in utero* were available. The fact that this has changed and that for some rare deformities fetal surgery is possible only intensifies those questions of "a social sort."

As a result of the counselors' invitation, I joined their workgroup. I attended

Chapter 6 was originally published as Charles L. Bosk, "Invitation to Ethnography," in *All God's Mistakes: Genetic Counseling in a Pediatric Hospital*. (Chicago: University of Chicago Press, 1992), 1–19.

preclinic conferences at which management of upcoming cases was discussed, observed the counseling sessions themselves, and listened to the counselors evaluate their work in a postclinic conference. In addition, I interviewed a sample of parents whose counseling sessions I had attended in order to gather their understanding of the process. Finally, I was on call for those emergency situations in which physicians in the newborn nursery or the neonatal intensive care unit needed to consult with the physicians specializing in clinical genetics.

The interactional data from my firsthand observations is the starting point for each discussion of shopfloor work. But to write of genetic counselors ethnographically is not to write of some tribe isolated in the bush, impervious to the wider world around them. Both genetic counselors and sociological observers who trail behind them need to take that wider world into account. Ethnographic descriptions of the applications of clinical genetics in the modern American hospital need to be mindful of the legacy of earlier attempts at eugenics, as well as the legal, political, and cultural questions that current practices raise.[2]

Starting with interactional data, the lived experience of patients and their doctors, I will move beyond thick description (Geertz 1973) to an analysis of what these patterns of interaction say about role systems, their domains, and their boundaries; about areas of collective consensus, uncertainty, or confusion; and about the policy alternatives we face as a collectivity.

An Invitation to Fieldwork

I was invited into this setting as a guest of the genetic counseling team because of their sense that as a sociologist trained to observe behavior as it naturally occurs, I would have something useful to add about how best to manage the myriad of social problems that trailed in the wake of new clinical developments. Since professional groups so rarely invite study by outsiders, it is first necessary to comment, albeit briefly, on this invitation and its implications for the ethnography before moving on to the substance of the text.

I received this invitation because I am a medical sociologist, an ethnographer of medical action. Here it is worth mentioning that today I would be unlikely to receive such an open-ended invitation. Since this fieldwork was done, formal institutions (ethics committees) and workers (bioethicists) have emerged for managing precisely the types of issues that the genetic counselors wanted help with. Back then, it was not so, and the help of any ethnographer was sought. By any technical, formal, scientific criterion, my data-gathering techniques are primitive, crude, and inevitably interlaced with my own subjectivity. I observe patients, physicians, and nurses as they go about the business of being ill, curing, and caring. My data comprises the behaviors I observe, the conversations I overhear, and the responses to questions I am not too timid to ask. At a phenomenological level alone, being a medical ethnographer is a peculiar occupation. For example, fieldwork on a genetic counseling service involves repeated voluntary participation in and observation of many of life's most awful moments, watching others cope with what the genetic counselors, ruefully echoing those who seek their services, refer to as "all God's mistakes."

However odd the work, anthropologists in the bush and sociologists on urban streetcorners have made ethnography a familiar mode of academic discourse. For the ethnographer in a medical setting, health-care workers are an exotic tribe; the bounded whole of the modern hospital is the bush. Our task is to rèport on the goings-on in this faraway province. At worst, we are voyeurs whose reports are a source of academic cheap thrills; at best, we are witnesses reporting on the most profound dilemmas of the human condition.

Not surprisingly, I prefer the latter self-description. As witnesses, we have two objectives. The first is to provide an empirically thick description of what happened: who did what, to whom, in what circumstances, with what responses from others, to what end, and with what consequences. The second is to analyze this description of the everyday, ordinary business of being a provider or consumer of health services. We inspect the record, as it were, for the evidence it contains about what it means to be a person, a family member, a citizen in modern American society.

As a witness in the arena of everyday medical life, as a sociologist, my perspective is explicitly dramaturgical. I think of clinical action in terms of situations—in particular those in which clinical action is problematic. Procedurally, I examine these situations to uncover what rhetorics, rationales, maxims, myths, data, and bottom lines physicians arm themselves with when they recommend one course rather than another to patients, when they explain unexpected, unwanted outcomes, and when they search for reasons to explain pain and suffering.[3]

As a medical sociologist/ethnographer, I have spent time in a variety of settings. However the settings varied, the central feature of my work as a sociological ethnographer remained the same. Data were generated by my skill at manipulating my relationship with my subjects. Invariably, and at one level, ethnographers treat their subjects simply as means to the end of generating good data on how some intractable problem of the human condition is managed among a group of natives.

Ethnographers—to the degree that they think about this practice at all—justify it by sleight-of-hand. It is not particular people that we are interested in, but general types, diffuse social and institutional processes, or native understandings. If people are treated as a means to an end, it is not qua people, but as mere representations of categorical schema. In presenting data, we do not betray individual trusts and confidences; instead we generalize them.

Most fieldworkers are not invited into medical settings; they are more commonly self-invited guests who find themselves backstage in medical arenas after complex negotiations to win institutional sanction. Most contemporary accounts of doctor-watching offered by sociologists stress the difficulties in gaining access to the private arenas in which medical activity takes place and in gaining the trust of physicians and other medical personnel. Fieldworkers invest the medical profession with many of the features that the nineteenth-century German sociologist Georg Simmel attributed to secret societies; then they describe themselves as minor Promethean figures eager to snatch secrets and place them in the public domain. In the most vulgar of fieldwork imagery, the medical profession is a living, breathing exemplar of G. B. Shaw's famous "conspiracy against the laity." The sociologist's task is to expose this conspiracy for what it is—the exploitation of pain and vulnerability for profit.

In characterizing the relations of doctors and patients, conflict is the social process and hostility is the emotional tone that are most frequently highlighted. Most medical ethnographers heed Hughes's (1971) injunction to study the "rough edges" of medical practice, those areas where lay and professional expectations about what action is necessary are least likely to converge. It is tempting to interpret this focus as the result of the difficulties experienced in gaining access to the fieldwork setting.

But what happens when such resistance is absent? What happens when the fieldworker does not worm his or her way into a site to pursue a personal agenda, but is invited in by physicians who have their own version of what the ethnographer's task is and what it ought to be?

Most practically, I experienced none of the difficulties associated with gaining entrance to the field setting. There were no negotiations with hospital administrators, no multiple clearances from multiple clinicians, and no endless rounds of meetings to explain who I was and what I was about. I was never asked to make elaborate promises to safeguard the confidentiality and anonymity of the institution or its physicians. Never was there any suggestion that my work be subject to any sort of prepublication preview. I had to obtain the official approval of an institutional review board, but that had more to do with government policy toward research subjects than with physicians' distrust of fieldworker sociologists. Moreover, as we shall see, I was asked by counselors on numerous occasions not to gather a consent but, nonetheless, to be in attendance.

Pilot observations began before the institutional approval was granted. Beyond that, the genetic counselors had been observed regularly by social scientists long before I got there. In the previous year, four graduate students had done fieldwork projects; one faculty member in the law school came to clinic and conferences quite regularly; and finally, a fifth graduate student was making observations preliminary to a dissertation proposal. At the same meeting at which the group asked me to join them, they worried out loud about "chronic crowding and being overstudied."

Of course, the absence of obstacles, as well as the plethora of observers, spoke of the desire of genetic counselors to receive sociological help. Their invitation to me was yet another artifact of their desire to provide their services as sensibly as possible. When they approached me, genetic counselors were aware that they were providing a new clinical service that intersected with some highly charged areas of social life, including the nature of parenthood and family bonds, and the permissibility of, and limits to, an actively preventive eugenics. In addition, the genetic counselors stated that there "were bound to be other difficulties that they could not foresee."

They asked for my help, which they envisioned as taking two forms. First, I could perform a hard-headed, objective assessment of how they were managing problems. In addition, I could provide a catalogue of the typical problems that they face but lack adequate resources to resolve. In accomplishing the first task, I would serve as an efficiency expert for the genetic counselors, providing data which allowed them to improve the quality of their services. In accomplishing the second, I would be a "committed moral entrepreneur," providing the society at large with data that would confirm the need to commit an even greater supply of resources to genetic counseling.

The genetic counselors believed that such a commitment was necessary and that, if I came to know their world as they did, I too would find such a need inescapable. This expectation—that our sentiments and analyses of societal interest would prove to be congruent—was, of course, unstated at the outset. It came with the invitation, but I did not realize it at the time.

At those early meetings, I was most struck by the counselor's recognition that the application of genetic knowledge in clinical situations created problems and that an interdisciplinary effort was called for to resolve them. I eagerly accepted the counselors' invitation, unaware of the implications of being invited to join the team—unaware of the difference between being an invited guest and being, as is more typically the case for a medical sociologist, an uninvited, albeit tolerated, intruder. Flattered by the idea that I might be useful, that I might have something to offer, I was seduced by the idea of pseudo-colleagueship. Not aware of the way this invitation, which amounted, after all, to nothing more than an opportunity to be an unpaid consultant, was a subtle devaluing of social science expertise, I joined the group. I joined unmindful of the consequences that belonging might have, first for observation, and later for reporting.

Invited Guests and Uninvited Intruders

If invited guest/uninvited intruder was a status distinction of which I was initially unaware, I quickly learned many of its nuances. In previous work, I had been an uninvited intruder (Bosk 1979). As such, I felt no special loyalties to the groups that I studied. I felt all the ordinary social constraints to treat them and their world with decency and respect, but I also recognized that in the course of things, I would bruise their cherished notions of their own goodness. But that was all part of making the latent manifest, of looking at social life unsentimentally, of revealing what goes on backstage. It was a part of all the formulas that sociologists have constructed to describe the unique perspective on the human condition that ethnography provides.

As an uninvited intruder, my relationships with my subjects were complex. On the one hand, in my day-to-day interactions, my subjects had no expectations of me. I was ornamental, decorative, extraneous, and dispensable. If I kept out of the way, if I was marginally helpful, if I filled rare downtime with interesting talk, whatever I wrote later was my own business. On the other hand, I was constantly tested, made the butt of group jokes, and accepted very slowly in the setting. What is critical is that whether I was an object of disinterest or suspicion for my subjects, I was expected to contribute nothing fundamental to the ongoing life of the group. When I did help, when I opened packages, passed supplies, or was simply an extra pair of hands, it was a welcome surprise to the surgeons. Expectations were low, and satisfying them was easy.

This was not the case when I was an invited guest. The genetic counselors had invited me to observe because they thought that I might help them. This expectation to be useful was unfamiliar to me. At case conferences, I was asked to provide concrete data about such things as how class differences or family structure affect patient understanding. I was asked to speculate about the handling of cases—to participate in the making of policy. How should couples who come in for sex selection be treated? What should the center's position on counseling for exposure to Agent Orange be?

Most frequently, the counselors asked for help on a range of clinical management issues: what social information to collect routinely for genetic registries, how best to give incoming patients reasonable expectations about their upcoming visit to the genetic counselor, how to avoid no-shows on clinic day, how to decide which patients needed which level of follow-up care, and so on.

> It is Friday afternoon, late in the fall. I am sitting, as I do every Friday after-noon, in a conference room for the postclinic wrap-up session that members of the genetic counseling team hold to report on their counseling sessions. Al Samuels (all names have been changed) is reporting on a case. Samuels characterized the session as "strange." He could not get a "fix" on whether or not the couple understood what he told them.
>
> He emphasized that they appeared to take everything in, yet as the in-formation got worse and worse, their affect did not change. Samuels giggled nervously as he concluded.
>
> Berger, chief of the Service, asked Samuels if he knew the parents' jobs. Samuels did not. Berger was displeased. He told the group that this was "stan-dard medical information which should be on record." He added a sentence or two about the importance of this kind of data, and the group moved on to discuss other cases.
>
> When the meeting broke up, I found myself going through the doorway with Berger. He led me a few paces away from the rest of the group and said, "I wish you'd push a little for medical records to include more social information. When I do, I sound just like a mother hen. But you, because you're a social scientist, perhaps you could get the others to see how important it is."

It was, of course, Berger who had initially invited me to join the work-group. Here was a direct example of him telling me how he expected me to be useful, what he wanted me to do: Be a missionary for social science data on medical records. Other members of the team also felt entitled to make special requests of my services as an observer.

The Mulroneys are coming to clinic for counseling.[4] They have a child with tuberous sclerosis. Mrs. Mulroney is pregnant. All the members of the counseling team save Berger are convinced that Mr. Mulroney has an extraordinarily mild expression of tuberous sclerosis. Berger is convinced that Mr. Mulroney is normal, and to the horror of the group, he intends to counsel the couple that they are not at any increased risk for having an affected child.

Bill Smith calls me at my office. "Bosk, you comin' to clinic?" I tell him I am. "Good, we want you to sit in on the Mulroneys and tell us what Berger says. We all think he's close to a serious error. But he won't listen to anybody. We want to know what happens."

This request—to monitor a colleague—was the most frequent special request that the counselors made of me. I was used in this way quite often when there was disagreement at Wednesday's preclinic conference about how to counsel the cases coming in that Friday. Not infrequently, I would be asked in postclinic conference if preclinic understandings were implemented, although never so nakedly as that. More often, it was just a vague invitation to talk: "Bosk, what did you think of the session?"

Conventionally, the sociological literature on fieldwork instructs us to turn such special requests and demands into occasions for educating our subjects about what fieldworkers do, or to volunteer just enough to get subjects to reveal their own feelings. The latter is a standard method for generating good field data.

With the genetic counseling team, neither approach was totally satisfactory. Didactic lectures *in situ* about the ethnographer's code of conduct and the importance of not interfering unduly with naturally occurring phenomena did not appear to be an adequate response to people who asked me to watch their work so that I could help. Moreover, even if I had wanted to help (and I am not certain that I did), more often than not I did not know how.

Called on often by the genetic counselors, I found that I had nothing particularly useful to say. Yet those invited to social occasions have obligations that those who merely intrude on them do not. As someone watching genetic counseling under the guise of having something instantly useful to offer, I often felt like a fraud when I let my hosts down by failing to meet their expectations.

I mention this because we shall see that my major criticism of the genetic counselors is their failure to be useful, to meet the patient on the patient's own ground, and to address the patient's most pressing concerns. The counselors, I will argue, at times use the goal of patient autonomy as a ground for patient abandonment. Sometimes, I wonder how much this insight grows out of my own sense of frustration at not being able to help the counselors more with applications of my specialist's knowledge in those very difficult situations where my help was requested.

With this example, I wish to call attention to a similarity between the work of physicians and the medical sociologist who trails behind them. The work of both involves explaining imponderables, and the failure to do so occasionally feels like a failure to meet a moral obligation. This example is a miniparadigm of how I was taught to act as a fieldworker, to use my own responses in a situation as a guide to the responses of others.[5]

I have mentioned that I thought the genetic counselors used the ideal of patient autonomy as an excuse for patient abandonment.[6] This is a sharp criticism, and since sharp criticism is often socially unpleasant (the essence of sheer effrontery), such sharp criticisms present a special problem to those invited into fieldwork settings: how to voice them in a way that does not give offense.

To use a social analogy, I was often in the position of the guest invited for a dinner where the experience of the meal itself is the entertainment—a feast. For this guest, nothing has been spared. The host has set the table with the best cutlery and china, given great attention to the menu, used the finest ingredients in preparing the dishes, and, nonetheless, produced an indifferent meal.

The guest is acutely aware of the meal's shortcomings; the host, however, is proud of his or her best effort. The meal consumed, the host turns toward the guest and awaits some comment. The host may grow anxious and fish for a response. The guest needs to find a way to respond to the feast that balances gratitude with honesty. That was my problem.

As hosts, the genetic counselors were unfailingly gracious. They offered me access to situations so acutely private that I sought rationales to limit my access. Gracious as hosts, the counselors were also anxious. They were constantly soliciting my evaluation of the fare they had placed before me.

Situations in which I had nothing to add presented me with one type of problem. My silence on troubling questions for me marked my failure to meet the moral and social obligations of the occasion to which my hosts had invited me. Situations where negative commentary was unavoidable presented another. What was the best response, if a commentary was requested, when I felt (as was most rarely the case) that the counselors had badgered their clients, or (as was all too often the case) when I felt that counselors had abandoned their patients by evading the real patient issues?

On the one hand, I did not want to insult my hosts' hospitality. On the other, I did not want to respond enthusiastically to dismal fare, only to see it served up proudly on all occasions. What did I owe the genetic counselors as a result of the unique field opportunity that they afforded me? At one level, I felt that I owed it to them to present my written criticisms at a very high level of generality, so that it was not individual counselors that I was criticizing, but the structural arrangements of care and the organization of social roles. But this satisfies the social obligation at a great remove from the time when it was actually incurred. How in the everyday context did I mix candor and kindness to respond to the needs of the genetic counselors?

The Witness Role

If I could be neither a garrulous nor an enthusiastic guest, in the spirit of the genetic counselors' invitation to join their team, what role then did I come to play in my three years with the counselors? How did I balance the genetic counselors' expectation that I be useful with my own methodological determination to remain detached and objective?[7]

I defined my work in two ways. I watched doctors with a well-defined set of sociological purposes at hand. I watched them to learn about the doctor-patient relationship, the division of labor, and the management of risk in the academic medical setting. But I also witnessed for doctors, and this witnessing for doctors was a more complicated business than ordinary sociological watching.

During the time I observed them, the genetic counselors faced many of the dilemmas that have become so familiar in the bioethics literature. For example, on several occasions the genetic counseling service debated whether children with trisomy 21 should be allowed to die from repairable defects; decided how the marginally competent mentally retarded should be presented with their reproductive choices; discussed whether parents were under any obligation to abort defective fetuses; speculated upon whether surrogate motherhood was a permissible remedy for certain forms of infertility (this well in advance of media disclosure and judicial notice of the practice); and tried to formulate cases under which amniocentesis for sex selection was ever acceptable practice. And this is only a partial list.

On many occasions, I was present not by chance but because my presence was specifically requested. Like the witness to any ceremony, my attendance was supposed to act as some sort of guarantee that proprieties were observed, that patient rights were respected, and that all the acceptable alternatives for resolving a problem had been explored. At the same time, I was a witness to the pain and suffering of patients as well as to how seriously the counselors took that pain and how hard they worked to mitigate it.

What separates witnessing for doctors from merely watching them with some well-directed set of academic purposes at hand is this: Witnessing seems more directed to establishing or ratifying a moral community than mere watching. Over time, I came to realize that not only did I witness for a group of physicians, but that those physicians did precisely the same for their patients. They listened to their patients' pains and problems, and the fact of the listening confirmed that the suffering was real and legitimate. Providing a place far from neighbors, friends, and family for couples to talk with specialists was all by itself something of a service.

Hearing a physician raise the option of artificial insemination by donor as a way to lower the risk of recessive disorder, or hearing a physician raise the possibility of institutionalizing a profoundly retarded child or discuss the possibility of abortion after a positive amniocentesis did not mean that the couple would necessarily rush to utilize these options. But it did mean that they had permission to think about them and that to do so was not necessarily immoral. If they did not do anything specific for a patient's pain, genetic counselors, at the least, gave them a place to take that pain; gave them "frames" and supplied "options." Given the shame and guilt that often accompany the birth of a damaged child, this was no small thing. Counselors then witnessed the pain of patients, and I witnessed the pain of counselors as they came face to face with their limitations in palliating the pains of their patients.

In a curious way, I came to symbolize for the group the moral community outside the hospital—my presence in highly problematic situations became a sign of approbation from the larger community of whatever course of action was taken. At one level this exacerbated my difficulties in giving the group negative feedback, but it resolved them at another. In any situation, I could simultaneously provide criticism and provide myself distance from it.[8] I would routinely speak not as an observer, but for some identifiable segment of the community and raise my objections in a voice that did not seem to be my own. I would begin most negative commentary by saying, "If I were a . . .", thus separating myself from my spoken words.

When the fieldworker is invited to join a medical team, witnessing is part of the fieldworker role at three different levels. First, at the simplest level, the fieldworker provides counselors with a "reality check," a confirmation that things are or were as they seemed. As a mundane example, whenever the genetic counselors described to others cases that I had observed, they would pepper their accounts with asides to me such as "Isn't that right?" or "That's what happened, isn't it?" Just as often, this confirmation was of the "God, did you see that?" variety; I helped make the incredible credible.[9]

Second, and unbeknownst to me at the time, a fieldworker, especially one whose presence has been requested, provides his subjects with a sense of legal protection. Being used this way happened to me late in my fieldwork, long after I had built upon that initial but shallow trust that the genetic counselors extended with their invitation to observe. Rather commonly, I found myself being asked to observe cases which were complex and contested morally, bureaucratically, and legally. I was on a number of occasions asked to observe as a "working" member of the team, to forego obtaining an informed consent from subjects, and to desist from public note-taking. While it would have been both ethically safe (and correct) to refuse such offers, the actual situations, along with their attendant negotiations, were more complex than that. Did a refusal mean that I was unwilling to act as a member of the team? Did the counselors have the right to seek my aid this way? Did I have a duty to refuse?

The compromise we arrived at was to have me introduced as a sociologist working with the team. I did not take notes at the time of observation, but wrote the cases up from memory. When a lawyer came to gather data for a wrongful life case, whenever a couple sought amniocentesis for sex selection, whenever parents sought to withdraw treatment from neonates, the group could press me into service as a team member. I slowly came to realize—slowly, perhaps, because I was gathering such good data—that the genetic counselors expected that should the need arise, I could serve as an expert witness capable of stating what had really happened. I do not know why the discovery of this latent dimension of my fieldworker role surprised and disturbed me, but it did, despite the large role that expert witnesses play in the civil procedures of the society.[10] Moreover, I shared with my genetic counselor subjects the feeling that being called into service as a witness in this way was annoying and burdensome.[11]

Witnesses play a religious role as well. Like the rabbi at a slaughterhouse, the priest at an execution, or the airline chaplain who consoles those awaiting passengers on a flight that has crashed, they purify and sanctify messy situations. In allowing me to view their uncertainties, anxieties, and doubts, the genetic counselors had allowed me to see their group function in an intensely religious and spiritual way. In hearing the genetic counselors discuss birth, life, and death, the boundary between them, and the permissible limits of human intervention, I was a witness to the group's "collective meditation on sacred things." For those social scientists who take their Durkheim seriously, such a meditation is the essence of religious experience. As such, it tells something of what these medical professionals hold sacred.

As I have stated, the genetic counselors were all too aware of the ways in which the organization of genetic counseling might disturb lay sensibilities. Having as their only treatment recommendation second-trimester abortion, and practicing in a society where the right to perform this procedure was a hotly contested political issue, they could scarcely avoid the ethical tensions created by their work.[12] When most aware of these tensions, the counselors often tried to draw me into their deliberations as a medical ethicist. I invariably demurred when called on to act in this way. I mention this now only because my silence on matters of medical ethics as they unfolded in clinical situations is in such sharp contrast to my volubility in the pages below, which are so far removed from the contexts in which words might have been helpful.

Soft Data, Hard Problems

I also mention my silence regarding medical ethics because if fieldworkers' canons of methodological purity commit them not to act as situations unfold, then it seems fair to ask just what do they contribute; why are they there, and are they necessary? Most simply, fieldworkers watch, listen, and use their own feelings and responses as guides to their interpretation of what is going on. In essence, this kind of observation is not terribly different from what psychiatrists, psychologists, and social workers are instructed to do as therapists. As Geertz (1973, 26) points out, ethnographic knowledge shares much with clinical inference.

The uniqueness of the fieldworker role comes from how that observation is used. Therapists are urged to use their feelings, instincts, and observations as a guide in responding to clients. For the therapist, for almost all those that use the logic of clinical diagnosis, the witnessing of action is a prelude to activity. This is true for other routine witnesses in the society as well, such as beat policemen and judges, basketball referees and baseball umpires, disability review panels and insurance adjusters.

This is not so for the fieldworker, who absorbs but does not respond to the situation. The task of the fieldworker is to witness again and again, but not to use the data gathered this way in interaction. Rather, the fieldworker observes to write. Patients, doctors, and most every other native ever observed write as well. But unlike fieldworkers, they had to act; the fieldworker has only to observe. This freedom from intervention and from ordinary interaction allows fieldworkers their special purchase on social life.

Gusfield (1981) speaks of this purchase as an Olympian one. The image better describes the aspirations than the accomplishments of fieldworkers: namely, to describe without sentimentality the way the world works. The ethnographer produces a social description, which is an imaginative construct. This description unpacks the interlinkages between everyday understandings, power, authority, and routine social action in revealing why things are as they are. In addition, as Gusfield shows so masterfully in his analysis of drinking and driving, such a description provides a glimpse at alternative constructions of the social world.[13] Once the world is imagined in this way, it can be imagined differently.

But what do sociologists as fieldworkers uniquely contribute to public life by imagining the world differently? This question has no simple answer. But if we return to the case of genetic counselors, we can provide a rough outline of the major dimensions of any adequate response to the question.

First, fieldwork alone places us in primary contact with social life as it is lived. The pains, the pressures, the perils, and the pleasures of the genetic counselor's work as well as the sorrow, shame, and existential guilt of parents are apprehended as they unfold in context, or are later commented on in soliloquies.[14] Fieldwork allows us to describe a set of fundamental life experiences as they occur—it provides us with words to inscribe the arc of human experience. In a field like genetic counseling, where the underlying technology threatens to revolutionize medical practice, it allows us to see the embedded tensions that lie beneath the surface of a rapidly advancing and dazzling medical technology: What is help? How is it provided in this society at this time? Fieldwork supplies precisely what other research methods drop out—the experiencing individual as a member of a community and the set of shared meanings that sustains that individual's action in an uncertain world. Fieldwork allows us to describe social life as we live it.

But that is not all fieldwork provides. It provides us with an opportunity not just to describe the lives we lead, but to analyze them. When it is performed with skill, it allows us to examine the shadow that falls between the image and the reality.[15] In the case of genetic counselors, this has meant matching counselors' statements about intent and purpose with daily encounters. For example, the counselors think of themselves as a support service, but then that support is most routinely defined as providing factually correct medical information.

Fieldwork, then, provides a mirror for looking at who we are, as compared to who we would like to be. It provides us with soft data: observations, intuitions, and comments for rethinking some very hard questions about what it means to be a member of the society.

Notes

1. The invitation to observe came in the spring of 1976. Preliminary observation lead to a proposal which was subsequently funded by the National Institute of Child Health and Development. The first period of intense observation began in the fall of 1976 and ended in the winter of 1978. In the winter of 1980, I reentered the field, only to leave again in mid-autumn of that year. My comings and goings were not random or unmotivated, but were rationalized theoretically at the same time that they were personally necessary. For now, that is all that needs to be said about the matter. The confessional of the fieldworker (Van Maanen 1988) is more appropriately an appendix to a text than a sentence in a footnote.

2. The introduction briefly considered historical antecedents of current attempts at applying genetic knowledge. In assessing current attempts at applied eugenics, we need to consider as well contemporary attitudes about risk, technology, the nature of birth, and therapeutic abortion. In trying to parse the current meaning of clinical genetics, the behavioral events observed have little meaning outside their arenas of production and interpretation. Some areas of genetics have become social problems, while others are relatively unproblematic. Understanding why this is so is a major task of the sociology of social problems (Hilgartner and Bosk 1988; Schneider 1985).

3. This paragraph is an echo of Garfinkel's (1967) charge for the study of social life in "What Is Ethnomethodology?" The echo is meant as a gesture of respect and a literal description of how I try to frame situations that are meaningful to me as a medical sociologist who works methodically as an observer.

4. For further discussion of the Mulroneys and their problems, see Bosk 1992, Chapter 2.

5. As a miniparadigm, it is a good example because it is so extreme, because it makes so much of the fieldworker's subjectivity, and because, like fieldwork itself, it is nonfalsifiable.

6. While I speak in this chapter about genetic counselors first and foremost, I do not feel that counselors alone are guilty of using autonomy as a warrant for abandonment. I am not singling out counselors as the solitary abandoners of patients amongst all the medical profession. Instead, I am using counselors to show how rather extensive patient abandonment can occur under the banner of more perfect patient autonomy. The very fact that counselors can abandon patients is noteworthy because it runs counter to so many elements of their occupational ideology.

7. Another old-fashioned aspect of this account was my determination to remain value-neutral. This is a role that both sociologists and anthropologists have long ago abandoned for a more forthright advocacy for the disadvan-

taged or paid consultancy for the privileged. Aware of the development of a more clinical sociology, I find it hard now to explain why I struck such a distant and remote definition of the task at hand.

8. For a full development of role distance and the repertoire of techniques that surgeons and teenage girls on carousels use to achieve it, see Goffman's (1961c) seminal essay. Here I am simply describing one ethnographer's ploy for achieving the same end.

9. Interestingly enough, I was used by surgeons in the same way. Some aspects of witnessing are built into the fieldworker role, whether the fieldworker is an invited guest or an intruder.

10. Fieldworkers have long worried about being co-opted by those that they study, and this worry is all the greater when we are studying up the social structure rather than down. Empathy with the wretched in society is rarely, if ever, considered a methodological problem. On the other hand, empathy with the powerful, with physicians, is seen as considerable cause for alarm. Here, though, I am fretting about more than where my loyalties lay. I am concerned about what my expertise is as well: what does it mean to represent oneself as "a skilled ethnographer"; what, save writing skillful ethnographies, can others expect me to do?

11. See Bill Smith's comments about being a witness in a wrongful life action (Bosk 1992, chapter 5).

12. The genetic counselors have much in common with the abortion counselors described so well by Joffe (1987). There is, however, this important difference: the abortion counselors were guided by rationales anchored in an applied social utilitarianism. The genetic counselors were also applied utilitarians, but they anchored their utilitarianism in genetic knowledge and paid virtually no attention to the social and economic contexts of pregnancy. For the genetic counselors, the only unwanted pregnancies were those planned pregnancies in which the fetus had an identifiable defect.

13. Gusfield's analysis begins by questioning our collective conventional wisdom; for example, the taken-for-granted assumption that reducing the number of individuals who drink and drive is a policy lever for improving highway safety. Why, Gusfield asks, does not the lever lie elsewhere? He then identifies a number of plausible alternatives to conventional wisdom: improved mass transportation, safer highway design, more crash-worthy automobiles, or a reduction of societal dependence on alcohol.

14. My collection of soliloquies is heavily skewed. I have a large collection of such asides delivered by physicians, but very few from patients. Part of the reason for this is structural: I was simply "backstage" more frequently with the genetic counselors than I was with patients. But while structure is important, it does not explain everything. I found my more private moments with parents, listening to their stories, painful. As a result, I did not do everything I could and should have done to expand my corpus.

15. This paraphrase of T. S. Eliot's "The Hollow Men" is used here with some trepidation. For all I know, Eliot felt, like Auden, that thou shalt not "commit a social science."

SEVEN

A Twice-Told Tale of Witnessing

I described earlier how I was invited to join the genetic counseling team, how I thought the invitation carried with it some vague obligation to help, and how I felt that I completely failed to meet that obligation. Then, in a manner surely different from what C. Wright Mills meant when describing sociological imagination, I made of my private troubles a public issue. I indict the genetic counselors for meeting client needs in a perfunctory manner. The fact that their work is anchored in a pediatric hospital allowed me to indict the entire medical profession for its inability to help those with intolerable troubles. I directed my attention to the "rough edge" of practice.

As a result, this account of workplace practices in a pediatric hospital virtually ignores the "smooth interface." I entirely fail to mention, or mention only in passing, that the limited goals counselors set for themselves—providing the most value-neutral assessment of conditional probabilities—was often what the person asking the question most wanted, whether that person was a treating physician or a lay service user. Rather than parading the countless examples of those occasions where genetic counseling, or the overall medical care of which it is but a small part, is a triumph of expectations fulfilled, I carefully dissect those occasions when genetic counselors, or others in the pediatric hospital where they worked, found themselves fre-

Chapter 7 was originally published as Charles L. Bosk, "A Twice Told Tale of Witnessing," in *All God's Mistakes: Genetic Counseling in a Pediatric Hospital.* (Chicago: University of Chicago Press, 1992), 160–83.

netically navigating a situationally stormy rough edge. Few if any "smooth interfaces" get displayed in typography that signals their status as relics from my fieldwork notebooks.

When the genetic counselors invited me to study them, it was with the expectation that I would produce a portrait, "warts and all." With ethnographic license, I produced one that looked only at warts. I have always assumed that such one-sided attention was necessary to construct ideal typical accounts of social process in bounded wholes, which is what I take the task of ethnography to be. With full ethnographic faith and self-confidence, I paid less attention to the fact that more than a single one-sided account is possible, or that my one-sided account might be unfairly distorted.

After all, a quite different account is possible. The genetic counselors could be just as easily described as heroic individuals able to suppress their own preferences and provide value-neutral statements of conditional probabilities. As experts, they do not let their values intrude on their professional/technical expertise. Approaches to care such as the counselors adopt reverse professional dominance in dealing with clients and avoid intraprofessional wrangling in the workplace when dealing with colleagues. Certainly the restraint of genetic counselors in the service of patient autonomy deserves more credit than it is given in the text.

There is another alternative. The genetic counselors are only "occasional" clinicians. Their limited patient-contact hours and responsibilities free them to meet research obligations and allow them to meet the demands of family life or pursue personal interests. The organizational niche of genetic counselors could have been presented as an attractive solution to the tension between the "greedy" claims of the service obligation and those of self, family, and community (Coser 1974). The boundaries that genetic counselors place around their involvement in clinical activity could have been presented as an ingenious tactic for preserving a personal self in a professional occupation (Zerubavel 1979; Broadhead 1983; Gerber 1983).

I also never stopped to worry that some of the data might have been gathered unethically. After all, I sometimes lacked fully informed, voluntary consent. While genetic counselors volunteered for study, other pediatricians were observed without their knowledge, as were patients; when consulting, there sometimes was not ample opportunity to introduce the ethnographer. If opportunity existed, it was hard to imagine at the time how the introduction would help a troubled situation.

Two instances of ethnography without consent are prominently displayed and analyzed in the text. Neither Doctor Marceau nor the Doughertys (Bosk

1992, Chapter 3) had any idea who I was as I sat next to Bill while they had their options conference. I note in my description that Bill is angry at Marceau but fails to say anything. Like Bill I was angry too. I sat silent as a stump. A question from me would surely have remedied the defect in care that the text complains of. How can I tell this story now about "using didge and diuretics to let nature take its course" if it fails the most basic ethical muster for research? This is guilty knowledge. Is there any benefit to telling the story? Could there be any harm?

I also lacked fully informed, voluntary consent in both Baby Doe cases, though in slightly different ways. I had an open invitation to attend weekly clinical genetics rounds. The first day I attended was the day that "the baby" in Chapter 4 of *All God's Mistakes* was discussed. People spoke freely and learned later that a witness was recording their words. In the second case, I was someone who came to a conference about a case whose management had troubled the pediatric staff. The purpose of the meeting was to air those differences and leave them behind. In such meetings, the ethnographer retrieves what the workgroup wishes buried. I was at a public meeting at which the public understanding was that there would be no public record. I have created one. Did I have the right to do that? Does the hiatus in time between collection and the breach of confidentiality mitigate at all the absence of consent? Does consent matter in ethnography? How?

In this chapter, I want to return to my self-casting as a witness, but this time in terms of tensions I felt as I collected data. I want to recapture the decisions I made along the way about what to observe, what to notice, and what to present. In addition, since I located my analysis in my own sense of powerlessness when called upon by the genetic counselors to help, I need to describe here those situations in which the counselors asked for help and how I helped them or let them down.

Ethnography and Editing

Ethnography is an immensely selective description of social life. What we observe is always less than what happened; what our notes record is always less than we observe; what a book includes is always but the merest fraction of notes. Ethnographers need to analyze the materials they include in their accounts and need as well to say something of what they exclude.

Chapters 2 through 5 of *All God's Mistakes* concentrate on formal meetings between physicians and parents or among physicians and other health care professionals. Almost everything reported in the text occurs in an arena, or is an activity that has a formal name in the pediatric hospital. This is much more an account of what people did in public situations than what they privately felt about them. Where the text recounts private feelings, it generally reports on their expression in professional arenas (such as post-clinic conferences) expressly created for the purpose of airing those sentiments. The stress on professionally public arenas was one way for me to resolve both the objectivity and the consent problem. Even so, the ethnographic practice of using the best notes, the most dramatic cases, the most floridly described situations undermines the objectivity sought. Moreover, the ethnographic selection from fragments is inherently problematic, since the same fragments can be arranged into so many other alternative accounts. Beyond that, a multiplicity of alternative accounts lies buried in field materials not cited.

Fieldnotes are representative, but ethnographers choose what it is they represent. At any rate, there is an inherent tension between an objective, empirical, ethnographic description and sociological frames of reference committed to examining the rough edge, reversing conventional sentimentality, or more simply describing the "contestable" autonomy of parents, prospective parents, and physicians.

The fieldworker can do more, however, than formally describe an ethnographic database, a set of self-generated fieldnotes, and the principles by which they were manipulated. The ethnographer can try to explain what is no longer stored in the notes or memory, what is not available for latter analytic working over. Ethnographers like me have trouble enough making sense of what is in our notes. We are often overwhelmed by the intricacy of what we observed. But—the point warrants repetition—we need to think as well about what we did not see, or what we saw but omitted from our fieldnotes. If we let our data speak to us and only report what happened, there is much that an interpretative ethnographic account cannot offer. Structured silences[1] and baffling omissions are important. We have to learn to identify and interpret them.

Structured Silence in Fieldnotes

One active way I have found for doing this is encouraging those I observe to repair the silences that I notice and consider proper to ask about. I record both what the genetic counselors did and said and a great deal of their commentary on actions not taken. In my notes, there is a continuing conversation, mostly with Bill but with all the others as well—a conversation made out of my asking someone why they had done one thing rather than another. After a while in the field, the genetic counselors volunteered such explanations without my asking. In a spontaneous burst of talk, they would formally articulate their decision tree. I assume that all ethnographers have such conversations with subjects. We teach by our questions what we are interested in; our subjects learn what we are interested in and volunteer answers to questions unasked. Such questions are the fieldworker's equivalent to the genetic counselor's passing parents a karyotype: they are a knowledge template.

We explicitly ask about the structured silences and the baffling omissions of others. But what of our own? I found my fieldnotes empty in three places where I expected them to be rich with data. These are worthy of description and analysis.

CLOSET CONFERENCES

The text reports that the Delberts' (the couple with possible G-syndrome) counseling session was interrupted. I noted that such interruptions were frequent and marked for me how genetic counselors failed to provide, at a basic level, any counseling at all. I did not note, but probably should have, that the work team on clinic day viewed such interruptions very differently.

For them, they provided opportunities to help in "story repair" when proper examination exploded understandings arrived at during rounds, for gathering composure after a patient dropped a "bombshell" in a session,[2] for figuring out what to do with the unexpected couple who just showed up or with the edgy couple waiting with justifiable impatience for the colleague who had not yet appeared. The Delberts' interruption was one of the few times that I did not excuse myself and go with Smith, Samuels, or Giordano.[3] That fact explains why it is recorded in my notes. When I left, I didn't record it. So, although I am sure such interruptions were "frequent," I cannot prove it with the kind of evidence that I have learned to trust; it's not recorded in my fieldnotes.

One of the reasons that I am sure such interruptions happened frequently is that I remember so vividly where the impromptu consultations arranged at the price of interruptions occurred: the supply closet, which was really a treatment room too small for conducting an examination. I remember being frequently huddled in the closet with the group. But this is not in my notes either. Moreover, closet conversations were more frequent than interruptions. They could occur legitimately between scheduled appointments, before work began, and as it ended, before the fully assembled group trooped over to the official conference room in an adjoining part of the hospital.

Why are the meetings in this space never recorded? The omission is even more startling in an ethnography that claims expressly some linkage to the work of Hughes and his students. After all, the supply closet is the quintessential backstage as described by Hughes's student, Erving Goffman:

> Here the team can run through its performance, checking for offending expressions when no audience is present to be affronted by them; here poor members of the team who are expressively inept can be schooled or dropped from the performance. Here the performer can relax, he can drop his front, forget speaking lines, and step out of character. (1959, 112)

Ethnography is prized over other methods for its ability to go beyond understanding formal staged performances; it reveals the grimier backstage arrangements necessary for formal staging. It is the backstage that is the repository of prized knowledge about how workers feel about their work, how they understand what they are doing, and how they define what the right thing to do is, in any situation. Yet my notes are empty of closeted information. Why? I knew the conversations were important. How do I excuse their omission first from my consideration and then the reader's?

As a sociologist, it is easy here to fall into some variant of ecological determinism. Spatial arrangements made it impossible. It was a small supply closet; that smallness made unobtrusive note taking impossible. This tidy explanation overlooks the routine writing others did in the supply closet and the fact that I had no qualms about the obtrusiveness of my note taking in counseling sessions, where I scribbled furiously as genetic counselors and parents talked. In any case, not taking notes at the time does not explain why there is no mention in my notes of these conferences. Quite a lot makes its way into my fieldnotes that I do not write down at the time. As an ethnographer, I take some justifiable pride in my ability to recall insignificant details. So how could the workgroup's most routinized backstage activity fall out of this account?

This is partly a matter of manners. One of the first times that I participated in a closet conference, I was told and asked, "This kind of discussion has nothing to do with what you're studying, right?" I remember being evasive; offering reassurance but fully intending to gather as much of "that kind of discussion" as I could. But I did not. The genetic counseling group set some observational boundaries; as best I understood them, I tried to respect them. Subjects have privacy rights; determining their exact nature is difficult to do with precision.

Where this account provides backstage performances—Bill and Al's disagreement over who "wears the green suit" or the team's discussion of when patient decisions give one cause "to jump off a bridge"—I have breached that boundary despite notes that are the model of restraint. Keeping "supply-closet conferences" out of them is an index of that restraint.

BERGER'S DEPARTURE

The second structured silence of my notes involves Berger's passing from and Palmer's coming to the workgroup. One would think that such change in leadership would be a natural topic for a workplace ethnography. Berger was a figure who linked the "old" and the "new" Nightingale Children's Center. Nationally, Nightingale's standing in clinical genetics was clear: it was "Berger's shop." His departure itself was an early indicator of the passing of the first post–World War II generation of physicians from academic pediatrics. Berger had a general pediatrics practice, albeit a small one, as well as his counseling cases. He was a representative of the last group of individuals able to link the clinical side and the bench science. None of the others who acted as genetic counselors maintained any general pediatrics caseload, although Giordano maintained a large high-risk obstetrics practice. Berger's departure is an example of the growing distance between general and specialty practice at Nightingale Children's Center and other hospitals of its eminence nationally, as well as an indicator of how genetic counseling services were becoming part of standard obstetrical care.

But there is precious little of Berger's departure in my notes. In fact, my notes from the time Berger announced his departure until Palmer clearly had assumed his duties display a number of odd characteristics. First, the notes from this period are almost exclusively of who said what in counseling sessions or discussion of cases from conferences. Little talk that is off track is noted. Second, the notes themselves are somewhat more spare and unelaborated than notes taken earlier or later. For example, couples are very rarely described or even named, beyond "the couple." There is a remote mechanical feeling in all of the notes taken at this time. In addition, during the time of Berger's leaving, I made myself generally available to the work group. In fact, I had some need to be around them to listen and to talk. Berger was my patron too, in a loose manner of speaking—if not my patron, my elder. In the local community I grew up in, that counted for something.

So it was not the case that the genetic counselors did not talk about Berger's departure, nor that I made myself so scarce that I never heard them. In fact, I remember long talks within the group as a whole and with each individual about it. But Berger, with his invitation, had set a mandate: I was asked to study the problems of providing genetic counseling as a service. Clearly, the problems caused by personnel changes at Nightingale Children's Center and their consequences for health care were well outside that mandate.

THE PATIENT'S PERSPECTIVE

The third structured silence in my notes, unlike the other two, has nothing to do with my reverence for the sensitivities of those I observed. It has much more to do with the feeling that I could never shake that there was something mildly ghoulish about the inquiry I was conducting. The last structured silence in my notes involves the patient's perspective. I did not try to enter the patient's perspective as completely as I did with physicians.

During the "pilot" part of this research, Smith, Giordano, or Samuels asked the counselees if they minded "if other members of the group joined us for today's session." No "users of the service" ever said no. The genetics counselors exercised some censorship, steering me away from cases that were "inappropriate for an observer." Of course, those cases intrigued me the most. When the pilot project ended, a consent form was given to all those who came to clinic whom I was scheduled to observe. But the consent form did not hamper cooperation either. Only one person ever refused to participate in the study. She was right to refuse; she should never have been asked.

My notes do not record whether she was asked at my insistence over the genetic counselor's objection, or whether we were a collusive net—they might have wanted me to watch Samuels work. (The woman felt that her albinism caused others to think of her as "a freak.") As Samuels recounted the case, I remember thinking, "There's no way that that session would have gone as well had I been there."

This was a jolting realization, as was its logical extension that perhaps much of my critique of genetic counseling is nothing more than an index of the strength of observer effect. Perhaps the kind of candid dialogue between genetic counselors and their clients which I find missing is missing because no one talks like that in front of a stranger, an intruder into the meeting with the genetic counselors.

I did make some feeble efforts to understand the parents' point of view in greater depth. For a number of parents, I conducted formal interviews. I use some of this material in the text; but I never really learned to talk with parents, to draw them out. I was not comfortable listening to the details of their pain. When the study began, I did not have children; I was deaf to the meaning of the parents' stories. When I became a parent, I tuned out the parents. It was simply too terrifying for me to try to place myself in their shoes.

I had opportunities to become more involved that I declined. The couple whose husband had been exposed to Agent Orange tried to recruit me for some advocacy work. I declined, but only after I turned off the tape recorder and explored for a while what they wanted. Had I accepted, I might have become the kind of "maverick" that Brown and Mikkelson (1990) say is so necessary to get environmental influences noticed in the public arena. Another time, a couple who had come in for what the text speaks of as "routine bereavement counseling" (their child had died from Sudden Infant Death Syndrome, and they were seeking reassurance that its cause was not genetic) invited me to come to their support group to see more closely how parents come to terms with grief. Again I declined.

On the genetic counseling side, Nancy Thomas had made an effort to get me interested in the support groups that are organized around specific genetic conditions. I have a folder full of the *Trisomy 13/18 Newsletter*. It is full of proud parental letters, helpful hints and advice, and reporting of birthdays. The folder is one research lead never fully explored, never fully integrated into the analysis. Finally, I never responded to the urging of another genetic counselor at an institution other than Nightingale that I carefully observe a third genetic counselor at yet another institution who worked closely with patient advocacy groups—a role eschewed by the genetic counselors at Nightingale, but nonetheless an important one for medical professionals and an interesting one to medical sociologists.

Of course, some closer contact with parents was unavoidable. Asking if I might interview them, then probing them about the experience of having a child die, or their understanding of the genetics, or poking around for evidence of discord in families felt intrusive, especially without a previous relationship and no promise of a continued one. With parents, I tended to be a "sociologist collecting data" rather than a person talking to other people. This is not a research style I recommend, although it served my emotional needs well. I shielded myself from parents with an extraordinary amount of formal pretense, but there were some who occasionally broke through to me anyway:

> I had asked the Cranshaws if I might interview them. They had already signed
> a consent form. They asked what I was going to do with the interview. I said I

would answer but asked why they asked. Mrs. Cranshaw said: "Well, if someone comes in and starts asking questions, you want to know who they are, and you wonder why he wants to know these things. I mean, I thought maybe you're writing a book." I admitted as much, and Mrs. Cranshaw replied: "Alright, so we're kind of going to be exploited."

These were my sentiments exactly. I had trouble concentrating during the rest of the interview as they told the story of their child's death. Instead, I kept asking myself to what end did I choose to do this. My most persistent memory of parent interviews is of myself as a polite, soft-spoken, psychological terrorist, whose questions abraded the thin tissue of cover parents had been able to place between themselves and great pain. Moreover, this tissue was one which the genetic counselors treated with great delicacy. It was almost as if my interviews somehow violated the "informal working" procedures of the group I was studying.

I did not like doing this fieldwork. But beyond that, I wondered how Bill Smith and Al Samuels survived in a clinical context in which they saw routinely so much horror and had so few opportunities for clinical "coups" (Bosk and Frader 1990). Joe Giordano, at least, had the compensating heroics of his high-risk obstetric practice. But for Bill and Al, the positives were tragedy averted, which, while it is an accomplishment, is not one without its darker side. I remember once asking Bill how he functioned in the Nightingale environment, how he came to grips with all the "accidents" or "mistakes" that he saw.

> What you have to do is this, Bosk. When you get up in the morning, pretend your car is a spaceship. Tell yourself you are going to visit another planet. You say, "On that planet terrible things happen, but they don't happen on my planet. They only happen on that planet I take my spaceship to each morning."

I never got as good as Bill at spaceship travel, at seeing Nightingale as another planet. I never mastered the language of its people. One of the few things that ethnography can do is represent those who would otherwise go unrepresented in collective debate. I have failed to do this for those on the other side of the counseling relationship.

In earlier fieldwork, looking at moral agency and general surgery residents and attending faculty, I likewise ignored the patient perspective (Bosk 1979). There, where the patientwas anesthetized on the table, ignoring the

patient did not make much of a difference. In the context of genetic counseling, where decision-making responsibility rests not with genetic counselors
but with parents, or is contested because parents are thought to be tainted
fiduciaries for their children's "best interests," this exclusive focus on medical professionals is more problematic, if only because moral agency is so
much more complex.

I claim to have been a witness to the work of genetic counselors at Nightingale Children's Center, but this "witnessing" seems oddly pitched. I was
so much a participant in some aspects of the genetic counselors' work that
I never stepped back and took notes on them. But closet conferences were
fundamental to understanding how the workers understood their work. Further, at a time—the transition from Berger to Palmer—when the meaning
and nature of the work was being openly reappraised, and when the genetic
counselors told me something that was, as Bill would put it "not for public
consumption," or as Al, Joe, Mary, and Nancy might say "not . . . the kind of
thing I would say publicly," I censored my notes for them. But how and why?
Such material—background understandings and backstage performances—
is central to ethnographic portraits of professional workplaces. In addition,
a deep engagement with the point of view of the user of genetic services
was something I assiduously avoided. In effect, I am silent as a witness on
those matters where as an ethnographer, I might be expected to write most
forcefully.

Beyond that, is there not something hypocritical in trying to wrap these
observations with a Hughesian cloth? The words are there, the proper incantatory formulas—"dirty work and good people," "routines and emergencies," "the rough edge of professional practice," and "guilt-sharing and
risk-spreading devices"—but the spirit is all wrong. I shunned the humble
and hung with the proud. And I was never properly "unconventionally sentimental" (Becker 1970) with them.

Intimacy and Distance

While I was in the field gathering data, I heard Hughes comment on a paper
("If Simmel Were a Fieldworker") presented by Eviatar Zerubavel (1979).
Hughes, who was in the audience, suggested that the title was misleading,
that Simmel was an extraordinary field-worker, a cataloger of the variety in
"the intersection of social circles." One type that Simmel draws with some
care is "the stranger."

The stranger, as Simmel describes him, confronts, like the ethnographer, the "particular constituents and partisan dispositions of the group" with a distinctly "objective attitude." But that objectivity is quickly tested in the field. As Simmel notes, the stranger "who moves on . . . receives the most surprising revelations and confidences, at times reminiscent of a confessional, about matters which are carefully hidden from everybody with whom one is close."

Ethnographers enter the field as strangers, but they cannot remain strangers long, and they do not move on so quickly. Gathering data on a group's ongoing life by observations means entering the group's workplace. For me, this has always involved requests from the workgroup for help. Surgeons (1979) asked me to push chart racks, open "four-by-fours," or "shine that light over here." What I was asked to do rarely disturbed what I was watching. An exchange took place; they let me hang around, but I had to give menial help back. Menial help was always welcome. There was always more than enough scut work to do.

Genetic counselors also asked me to help, but the help requested was no longer so trivial. It very often involved serious professional business: "Talk to this couple for a while and see if you can get a fix on them"; "Watch Al handle this case, and make sure he doesn't steamroll the patients"; "Observe Berger because we are worried about what he is going to say." I never questioned the legitimacy of any of these requests, perhaps seduced by the idea that I had something valuable to offer in a clinical setting, even if I did not precisely know what that something was. The genetic counselors spoke to me as a member of the genetics counseling team; more important, I agreed to listen as a member of the team. How else to explain the nearness of being in the supply closet with physicians and the distance of interviewing patients with a formal interview protocol.

To this social distance add the formality of getting a signed consent and audiotaping an interview, and the discontinuities between the ways I know the medical professional's perspective and that of the user of medical services are quite striking. Moreover, I was not a neutral, a "stranger," to the users of service. I was just another white, male doctor in a tie asking questions and taking notes. So my interviews with ordinary lay users of services were not the transcendentally confessional experiences a Simmelian stranger/researcher might hope for.

As a member of the team, I had certain obligations. The first was immersion in team activities. Immersion was not difficult to sustain, since team activity was focused on weekly preclinic rounds, clinic, and postclinic conferences. At other times, Al Samuels was in his lab, Joseph Giordano was at his obstetrics practice, and Bill was on call at Nightingale. At these times, I was released from the yoke of team demands. I taught classes, read, wrote, did committee work—the banal dreary task of ordinary teaching, which corresponded to the clinical banality of genetic counseling.

There was one other weekly gathering at which members of the genetics team were present, but I chose not to attend it. This was the weekly amniocentesis meeting, a Monday-morning case conference chaired by Giordano. At this meeting, the genetic counselors were submerged within a larger obstetrical context in an urban academic teaching hospital. This was defined as an obstetrics rather than a genetics event. I accepted that explanation and stayed away. After all, an ethnographer must observe something rather than everything. Genetic counselors were part of my something; obstetrics was not.

Staying away lowered the demands of the fieldwork. The post-clinic conference ended late afternoon or early evening on Fridays. The amnio conference began at eight on Monday mornings. I could not tolerate the sense of "being captive" that being with the genetic counseling team at the beginning and end of each work week created. Had my threshold for contact been higher, I would have been in a better position to observe the ways in which routine genetic counseling was transformed into routine amnio (and now routine chorionic vacilli sampling [CVS]) counseling and how much of the work was absorbed into the ordinary structure of obstetric care.

Besides the obligation of immersion and the obligation to respond to requests for help, the group expected from me a certain amount of loyalty expressed as circumspection. This should not have been difficult to provide. After all, ethnographic ethics require confidentiality. Simply put, we do not gossip about our subjects, except for our formal presentations and publications. The genetic counselors' demand for loyalty was nothing more than the expectation that I would not tell tales, and as such, it was one common to all ethnography, one I was familiar with as an experienced field-worker. It was an expectation that was more easily breached than I realized.

When I got to clinic, Bill said he wanted to speak to me about a case. He took me into an examining room and immediately began to talk. He said that he had spoken to my "friend, Farley," and that he had said he had heard that he (Bill) was not too happy with the way the case of a lethal form of dwarfism that they had counseled together had gone. The clear implication here was that I was the one who had told Farley this.

I don't remember telling Farley that. I do remember discussing the case with him. I do remember his being unhappy that the mother of the child had felt that the damaged child was a punishment for an elective abortion that she had had at sixteen. Farley felt that Bill did nothing other than repeat the bare facts of transmission to alleviate the mother's guilt.

I do remember mentioning to Farley that I thought in general that Bill was uncomfortable with expressions of affect in those he counseled. Bill, I said, defined his job as merely disseminating factual information, which he believed would all by itself remove the psychological burdens of genetic defects for parents.

After I spoke to Farley, I asked Bill and Nancy Thomas about the case. They both said that the session had gone terribly. They each described the session as a "classic case" of a woman who was feeling punished for something she had done a long time ago.

I asked them both how they managed these feelings in the session. They mentioned that the pediatrician in the case had suggested that they suggest that the woman talk to her clergyman about it. They said that this was a strategy they avoided until they had an opportunity to "check out" how the clergyman felt about such issues—the last thing they wanted was the guilt being reinforced.

I had thought that I had been particularly skillful in this case at "triangulating," or collecting multiple accounts. Bill, it seemed, now thought less of my practice of my craft. I had trouble listening to Bill, had trouble keeping straight his actual words. I knew he was mad that I had discussed this with Farley. I knew I had been wrong to discuss the case at all with Farley. I was mad at myself. I was mad at Farley for using me to support his evaluation of the handling of the case. I thought he had projected his feelings in the guise of mine. [At any rate, it is one thing to break confidentiality; it is another thing to be found out.]

Bill told me "to be careful, that what happened, it wasn't good." But I already knew that. Then Bill announced, "Well, now it's aired and that's that." And indeed it was, in a way that mirrored the complaint itself. Bill had described what happened; but he did not offer me an opportunity to say my piece, nor had he commented on his feelings. His anger was value neutral and nondirective.

Then Bill invited me into his next case with him. A gesture, much appreciated, that showed that, despite my indiscretion and his scolding, we were still friends.

To underscore the invitation, he added that the case was "interesting."

"Why?" I asked.

He told me a story about a woman (the person we were about to see, in fact) whose husband had threatened to "kill her and her baby, just last week. The husband had been shipped off to a mental hospital in Florida." Bill presumed the reason for this was that that was where his parents resided.

I agreed that it did "sound interesting." We then negotiated about how interested I was allowed to be. I asked if I could tape the session. "No," said Bill, "it would be too much like giving the woman the third degree." I asked about an interview. "Inappropriate, given the circumstances of the case," said Bill. "What about a consent form?" I asked. Again Bill said no. I went along again, not voicing my own objections to this way of doing research.

This is a "confessional tale from the field" (Van Maanen 1988), quoted at great length because it is so instructive of both the strengths and weaknesses of this piece of fieldwork. I think now that I should have had it out with Bill over the consent issue. I believe that the failure to gain a consent was a frequent occurrence, especially when cases were defined as "interesting," but I did not keep a running record of this delict in my field notes. But every time I proceeded without a consent, I compromised the research in important ways.

I think I knew that this was so at the time; my notes indicate a running internal dialogue with myself over the issue, but never an open public one with the group. My hesitancy to do this, which eventually became my failure to do this, I can quite easily rationalize: The research began in a preliminary way, which established ongoing ways of doing things. When a formal consent requirement was instituted, I had already decided to concentrate my attention as a sociological ethnographer on medical professionals and their workplace definitions of proper action. To insist on consent now, when I had been welcomed as a team member, would have jeopardized my access by placing loyalties in question.

Moreover, I was acutely aware of how many researchers before me had tried to study this group and had been actively rebuffed or had decided that this was a game not worth the candle. But I had committed myself to the challenge, not just because I thought the then-practiced clinical applications of genetics were sociologically interesting, but also because I thought the team at Nightingale would allow me access to a range of problematic situations for which ethnographic descriptions would be "good to think with," a way of giving behavioral specificity to a set of "essentially contestable" concepts like *patient autonomy, treatment decision, private matter, random accident,* and *freak occurrence.* The genetic counselors provided me legitimate access

to the world of Nightingale. In exchange, I gave up my professional autonomy as a researcher to ask what I wanted of whom I wanted.

Staying away from patients had more or less been a condition of earlier research, so I underestimated its importance in this research. What I had not
factored in was that for most patients, only one visit with a genetic counselor
was necessary. In another setting, say the intensive care units studied by
Guillemin and Holmstrom (1986) or Zussman (1992), the absence of an initial introduction would not have been a fatal flaw. Over time, as patients and
families assimilated the culture and procedures of the ICU, the sociological
observer was seen simply as one more person with a vague task. While not
critical to care or treatment decisions in this setting over time, the ethnographer is available to talk, which has a value all its own.

In genetic counseling, however, my collusion with Bill, my not gaining a
consent when that was not only appropriate, but in fact required by a University Institutional Review Board (of which I was a member), shut the lay recipients of genetic counseling services out of the study. After all, having been
introduced as a member of the team, I could hardly approach people and
explain how what Bill or Al or Joe had said, by way of introduction, "wasn't
true," and that "I wasn't really a member of the team," and that "I wanted to
ask them about how they really felt and what they really understood about
the counseling session."

Further, not having my "outsider" status clarified up front effectively si-
lenced the participant half of this participant observer in two ways. First,
couples, if confused, if in need of another opinion, if struggling with the
medical professionals of Nightingale Children's Center and in need of an
ally, could never turn to me and say "What do you think?" At the time of the
fieldwork I thought of this as a benefit. It made me confident that there was
little "observer effect," that I had not disturbed the field I had set out to describe, that I had not produced an account of how I stirred the dust striding
into the field.

Now, with very great hindsight, it seems to me that more observer effect
would have produced more understanding, a deeper appreciation on my part
of the experience of the lay users of counseling services. For surely I would
have been asked questions by a lay user only as a last resort, after all other alternatives to put together a usable version of reality had failed. At that point,
I would have been able to pinpoint with some precision breaches and gaps
between professional practices and lay understandings. The words that lay
users of genetic services might have addressed to me had they been able, had
I an existence and identity apart from "team member," surely would have

pointed me toward the "rough edge of practice." It is not hard to imagine that interviews might have been more productive, had I appeared to be less a formal agent of the team.

Beyond that, entering any scene as an "unannounced observer" forced me into silences like the one with Marceau and the Doughertys, which were themselves more unnatural than the dreaded observer effect I so much wanted to avoid. Normally, I think that my own credentials as a student of social life entitle me to "identify group problems and suggest solutions for them," but by not claiming such an identity, I deprived myself of a voice. More a shadow than a witness, I could not transform myself into an ally or advocate. Feeling that I observed under false pretenses, I lacked the right to ask the seemingly innocent question or make the innocuous suggestion that might help a stalled group get from there to here.

When all is said and done, it strikes me as peculiar that at the same time when sociologists were touting clinical skills in organizational and management realms or were retreating from value neutrality and producing "advocacy ethnography," committed to privileging a particular political perspective, I should fashion such an oddly passive role for myself, one that would neuter my knowledge in this arena of reproductive decision making. I suppose it is quite possible that I was simply mirroring the nondirective ethos and value neutrality which we have seen were such important parts of the work ideology of genetic counselors, that I overidentified with them so completely that I overgeneralized their workplace ideology, bootlegging it into my discipline from theirs. It is also possible that I was responding to tensions I felt within the discipline of sociology concerning the production of ethnography. By staying silent, by remaining aloof, I was trying to guarantee an objectivity I felt would be shattered by more direct involvement. Finally, I suppose that the "witness" role I fashioned was a "guilt-shifting" and "risk-spreading" device. If I never volunteered suggestions, if I insulated myself from the possibility of being asked the horrible "What would you do?" question, then quite clearly I could not make a mistake. I could not overstep my bounds.

Whatever my motives at the time, I would never again be so passive in a piece of research, I would never again pretend I had so little to offer, I would never again delude myself into thinking that being a "witness" was enough. The next time, the point would not be to describe and interpret the world, but to change it.

And here, as an ethnographer, I am at sea. I do not know how to change it. Moreover, if the point of being in a situation is to improve it through some sort of directed action, which could be as incisive as a scalpel or as gentle as a question, then the activity is no longer "doing ethnography." It is incorrect to say that ethnographers burn out; instead, we become experts in substantive domains. With this expertise and some of its organizational and cultural accoutrements (titles, committee memberships, public forums such as rounds and case conferences) goes some obligation to speak clearly about ongoing cases. My "expert talk" as an ethnographer on a genetic counseling team structured my subject's notion of what I found interesting, what they should tell.

In this case, the genetic counselors talked with me often in a very backstage way. For the users of the service, I was a white, male professional doing "research." I was much too close to one part of the doctor-patient dyad and remote from the other. This caused a regrettable silence at times.

Here, There, and Everywhere

The question of whether to describe pseudonymnously or to correctly identify is both an epistemological and ethical question for ethnographers. To describe pseudonymnously would seem too willful a distortion of a very objective reality. What is more real than the proper names of people and institutions? A second defect of calling someplace real *Nightingale*, and of identifying a specific person with a fictive name is that such accounts of local culture scrub away the very details that make one local culture different from all the rest. If I were more committed to phenomenology, I might say that pseudonyms remove a place's "this-oneness": all those markers which make it unique. Pseudonyms, by the norms of science alone, should be disqualified, since they name both unreliably and unverifiably.

Moreover, the normal conditions that justify pseudonyms do not apply here, as one reviewer of the manuscript pointed out to me. The genetic counselors are not urban outlaws or political revolutionaries whose lives I might somehow endanger if the police or the government read my manuscript. They are physicians and other health professionals in a setting which has received no shortage of discussion. What is to be gained by pretending that "Nightingale" is not somewhere real? Who will be fooled anyway? Generally, pseudonyms are quickly decoded. Everybody soon learns that *Street Corner Society* was done in Boston and that *Experiment Perilous* was done across the river at the Brigham. Why play games? Why insist on Nightingale?

There are a number of reasons. There is, first of all, a question of form. When writing about such mundane matters as the organization of services in a pediatric hospital from the perspective of a team of genetic counselors, to name names is to overspecify. What is important is not the specific person who did something but the less personal rationales that supported the doing. Naming names places the emphasis on the specific and not the general forms of a situation. For journalists (Lukas 1991) and Bauhaus architects, "God may be in the details," but in doing ethnography, a more secular aesthetic prevails.

There is the question of preestablished agreements. One part of the informal, unwritten agreement that was struck to allow me to watch this workgroup so intensely was, "You can report what you want. But you cannot report specifically who and where." On the counselors' part this was a reasonable restriction to make, since it protected patient confidentiality. I assimilated the professional norm of confidentiality in a way that mirrors the text and the world: I distanced myself from service users. For the first summer that I made observations (June 1976), my field notes are ordered by cases identified by service user names. The longer I am in the field, the less frequently are service users identified by name. They all become couples, a she or a he with an occasional baby, girl, or boy. On my part, patient confidentiality was a reasonable thing to assure. I could not see then and I cannot see now why the cast of characters should be properly named.

In fact, I have never understood why anyone has ever suggested differently. In the innocent act of giving a place a pseudonym, we move from a world of specific occurrences, each happening for their own uniquely recurring reasons, to an ideal type of greater generality. There is something of trying to make the mundane grand in this: Yankee City rather than Newburyport, Massachusetts; Middletown rather than Muncie, Indiana. Pseudonyms are a rhetorical device to remind ethnographers of their native land that one does not use ethnography merely to produce a literal record of who said what to whom. Rather, one uses ethnography to produce a focused, analytic account about how some recurrent dilemma of social life is managed. Using pseudonyms, if it does nothing else, signals ethnographic intent, which is interpretive. Conversely, using real names signals an intent which is more committed to uncovering the single truth about X.

In this instance Nightingale Children's Center and its genetic counseling team have been created by me to describe how a set of workers with a service ideology which was committed to enlarging the autonomy of those who consult with them by using nondirective, value-neutral counseling techniques fared in one, admittedly not very representative, pediatric hospital. My intent was to have the cases presented serve as springboards for thinking about a set of questions which vex me still, even as I try to write a last word about them.

This research occurred somewhere; exactly where is important, but beside the point. Some places I could have observed might have been much better at meeting user needs; others worse. However, none might have been so generous as Nightingale and its genetic counselors at providing so much diverse clinical material, so many of the problems that bedevil the definition, delivery, and evaluation of care and service.

The specific instances of care and service presented here all occurred a long time ago. There has been much change in genetics and health care between the observation and the production of the text. Nonetheless, the core issues—the nature of and limits on lay and professional autonomy, the proper balance of individual and collective values in decision-making authority, the shadowy line between public and private domains—these have not changed, nor gotten easier to resolve, despite organizational innovations. This account points to some reasons why this might be so. By making someplace real into Nightingale, I intend to indicate just how general and widespread these difficulties are.

It seems to me that pseudonyms make ethnography possible in a context where the natives are likely to read and critique the analysis of their community, for the protection of anonymity allows subjects to participate in those small betrayals of one's intimates that make for such good data from the fieldworker's point of view. At the same time, the blurring of details at the margin, the changing of names and the like, provides subjects some deniability when a book makes its way back to the local arena on which it is based. In local communities, ethnographies of professional communities are read in the same spirit as any *roman à clef*. Ethnographers owe it to their subjects to make the decoding process as difficult as possible.

Notes

1. I am grateful to my colleague Renée Fox for the term.
2. An example would be the surprise announcement of pregnancy by a couple with very real risks.
3. If Berger were present, no interruptions were brooked. Berger considered them "unprofessional." My notes record few times when Palmer's cases were counseled at the genetics clinic.

EIGHT

Irony, Ethnography, and Informed Consent

Bioethical analysis can be made sharper if more attention is paid to the context of medical decision making, and ethnography is the ideal method for accomplishing this. Intellectual completeness and honesty—not to mention the self-reflexive dimension of ethnographic work itself—require that attention to the ethnography of medical ethics be matched by a reciprocal analysis of the ethics of ethnography.

That is the task of this chapter. In it, I first discuss some of the standard ethical dilemmas fieldworkers recognize as inherent in ethnographic methods. Here, I argue that the commonly rehearsed ethical dilemmas of fieldwork screen our attention from some more fundamental problems of fieldwork, especially when that work is among highly literate subjects within one's own culture. Then, using my own fieldwork among surgeons, genetic counselors, and workers in a pediatric intensive care unit as an example, I discuss these primary, and perhaps irresolvable, ethical problems of ethnography.

Such an analysis is necessary for two major reasons. First, it will avoid the inevitable disappointment that occurs when an idea is pushed beyond its serviceable boundaries. Ethnography—and other forms of social science research—have a place in bioethics. They are useful in providing answers

Chapter 8 was originally published as Charles L. Bosk, "Irony, Ethnography, and Informed Consent," in *Bioethics in Social Context*, ed. Barry C. Hoffmaster. (Philadelphia: Temple University Press, 2001), 199–220.

to some sorts of questions and concerns but not to others. It is important to be clear about these limits. Ethnographers need to take care not to promise, and bioethicists not to expect, too much from a labor-intensive mode of inquiry that is highly dependent on the individual researcher's subjectivity, sensitivity, and interpersonal skills; that is useful for describing social process in very specific circumstances but not for generalizing across settings; and that has no way to describe values and beliefs other than as reflections of socially structured interests with no independent ontological status of their own.

Next, traditionally ethnographies have been done by ethnographers who occupy specific niches in social science departments, have received training in concrete intellectual traditions, and have very definite value commitments regarding the purposes of their work. Bioethicists occupy different occupational roles, receive a different training, and possess, as a rule, different value commitments. How well these two distinct sets of roles, training, and value commitments harmonize is an open question. I argue below that excellence in one domain—ethnography—may make excellence in the other—bioethics—difficult, if not impossible. At the very least, the doctrine of "fully informed voluntary consent" requires that bioethicists be aware of the risks and benefits of embracing ethnographic research, in particular, and social science methods, more generally.

Throughout this discussion, I point out some pragmatic difficulties in either creating or using ethnographic accounts as part of the academic literature of bioethics or the public discourse of the ethical dilemmas of medicine. For the purposes of furthering a discussion of *ethics*, ethnography, despite its superficial allure, is not ideal. The description is just too detailed; and if it is not, then the ethnography is inadequate, an unreliable basis on which to found an argument. The goal of ethnographic analysis is not to clarify on which values action should be bottomed. Rather, the goal is to show how flexible values are, how the same values are used to justify a wide range of seemingly incompatible behaviors. But there are other reasons for ethicists to be wary of ethnography. A close look at the methods used to generate ethnographic data and to produce ethnographic accounts raises questions that suggest that these research tools have insuperable ethical problems in terms of informed consent and the preservation of confidentiality and anonymity. These necessary moral failings are built into the structure of ethnographic research. This fact might give the ethicist pause before using the insights generated by such suspect behaviors. That these problems are largely unacknowledged becomes clear when we review the traditional approach ethnographers take to the ethical problems that they recognize as part of their research methods.

Everyday Ethics of Ethnography

For its first sociological practitioners, primary observation of social life was not problematic either methodologically or ethically. In the sustained body of urban studies produced during the 1920s and 1930s, the sociologists of the Chicago School studied the city as "a mosaic of social life" (Park and Burgess [1922] 1967). A key advocate of this approach, Robert Park, a former reporter, emphasized in his programmatic writing the connection between the physical and moral space of the city. The early monographs that the Chicago School produced all tended to be structured along very similar lines—a "natural" area of the city is identified; the demographic, geographic, and economic features of this unique "ecological" niche are specified through summary statistics; and, then, on the basis of observation and in situ interviewing, the "moral order" of the "natural" area is described. None of the authors of these studies raise any questions about the observational data. Valid data required only an observer with a notebook.

Questions about ethnographic methods begin within sociology, like so much else, with the publication of the second edition of William Foote Whyte's *Street Corner Society* (1955). Whyte reports that when *Street Corner Society* first appeared in 1943, its commercial success was underwhelming. Brisk sales came only with the revised, expanded second edition, which includes a methodological appendix that explains how the research was done. There are a number of reasons why the second edition was so much more commercially successful than the first. In part, the new appendix makes for a more artful presentation and for a more "real" account. But demographic and cultural considerations played a role as well. When college enrollments began expanding, there was a need within sociology for an accessible text to engage students. Also, in the war years the concerns of *Street Corner Society*—the assimilation and resistance of the sons of Italian American immigrants to mainstream American society—must have seemed far away. Oddly, the passage of time allowed for the subject matter to become more timely. Finally, Whyte's themes resonated with many of the ongoing themes of the civil rights movement and permitted their discussion absent race, which, undoubtedly, must have made the discourse more comfortable for a while at least.

Since Whyte, such appendixes are a standard part of ethnographic writing—so much so that Van Maanen (1988) in his survey of ethnographic writing identifies them as a distinct subgenre that he labeled "confessionals." Although Van Maanen's label has a trivializing connotation—think ethnographers on Oprah or Sally Jesse Raphael—it is also surprisingly apt. There is a sense in which one thing that all ethnographers do in appendixes is ask their colleagues' forgiveness for various sins against method idealized. In Whyte's first-ever example of what was later to become so stylized, he described what over time became the commonly rehearsed issues of participant observation with their standard solutions. The most important of these are as follows: the difficulties of gaining entry to a setting, of winning the trust of one's subjects, of balancing obligations to competing groups within the neighborhood, of verifying one's own insights about what is going on, and of leaving the setting.

From Whyte's appendix, we learn of his settling into Cornerville; of his meeting "Doc"; of his continual struggles to fit into the alien neighborhood of Cornerville; and of his initial indifference, then his excitement, and finally his horror at voting numerous times in a local election. This last revelation is a touchstone for confessional ethnographic writing. Whyte reports being troubled by this ethical lapse only when threatened with public exposure and disgrace. However much Whyte strains to sound concerned by his ethical lapse, his account conveys nothing so much as his excitement at being accepted and trusted enough to engage in this conventional political petty larceny.

Although there are a number of things worth noting about this report of the fieldworker's dilemma, one thing that is not is its resolution: to follow local customs, to go native. In fact, examples of instances in which the researcher behaved in ways that violated his or her everyday norms are easy to multiply. It is hard to imagine how it could be otherwise. After all, sociologists report being drawn to settings "where the action is," and the scene of ethically problematic activities is just one such setting (Goffman 1961). This is as true of the street corner and its petty crimes as it is of the intensive care unit with its ineluctable treatment dilemmas. One could hardly study such issues if one responded moralistically—to learn about fences requires knowledge of stolen goods (Klockars 1974), to study youth gangs involves observing street violence (Sanchez-Jankowski 1991), to observe how welfare recipients get by on limited incomes means keeping an open mind about what officials label welfare fraud (Edin and Lein 1997), to study decision making in intensive care demands suspending judgments about how such judgments ought to be made (Anspach 1993; Zussman 1992), and to catalogue medical error from the physician's point of view asks that other points of view be submerged (Bosk 1979).

In fact, when ethnographers evaluate their behavior in the field, they rarely use an ethical yardstick. Instead, they use a pragmatic one. The question is not whether the act in question violated everyday norms. Rather, the question posed is: Did the questionable behavior contribute to doing the study? With this kind of moral accounting, most actions, however far beyond the pale they are, are justified easily. But there is something self-serving in this. Ethnography is not a carefully controlled clinical experiment; the fieldworker never knows for sure what the consequences of acting alternatively would have been, never knows if the boundaries could have been drawn differently. This mode of moral accounting does, however, draw attention to a central facet of being in the field: The pressure to fit in, go along, suspend disbelief, and discount one's own moral autonomy in the name of research is enormous and, perhaps sadly, irresistible.

Nowhere in the writing about doing the research is the pragmatic stance of the fieldworker and its distance from a moral one so clearly marked as in discussions about gaining entry. In appendical musings, ethnographers recount their worries about fashioning plausible cover stories to explain their interest and presence in a field setting. A good cover story provides an easily understood rationale, but is not so overly detailed that it distorts later responses, creating dreaded "observer" effects. Many discussions of telling cover stories have a "comical aspect" (for a good example, see Bluebond-Langner 1978). In the typical account, the fieldworker reports great apprehension, a carefully prepared speech clumsily delivered, and, finally, the irrelevance of both the worry and the story itself. In the end, entry and trust are negotiated and renegotiated over time. What matters is not what is said once and formally, but what is done repeatedly and spontaneously.

Drawing on my own experience, I would place very bold quotation marks around the word "spontaneously." When I am in the field, very little ever feels spontaneous to me. Rather, I am constantly calculating and weighing responses in terms of the kind of data they are likely to yield in both the long and short run. To be sure, this is an instantaneous calculation in which I am most probably frequently wrong. Nonetheless, my responses are based on this; they are calculations, not spontaneous expressions of my most authentic, innermost self. The very fact that this is so causes me to wonder if ethnographers' understanding of observer effects is not as self-serving as their rationales for norm violations. Ethnographers acknowledge that observer effects rarely can be gauged directly from firsthand observations. Ethnographers cannot make observations of how group members behave when the ethnographer is absent. Then, ethnographers argue that in the face of natural role demands and situational exigencies, observer effects disappear over time, are minimal, or both. This is an argument that has considerable appeal, allowing, as it does, ethnographers to discount any impact they might have had on that which they describe.

This is an argument in which I once fervently believed—but lately, like some turn-of-the-century cleric exposed to Ingersoll, I have come to have my doubts. As I look over what I have observed, thought I understood, and interpreted authoritatively, I wonder how much was staged for my benefit. I have been blessed and cursed with "theatrical" natives with more than enough savvy to figure out my interests. Those disciplinings that modeled the surgical conscience (Bosk 1979), and those tortured, quasi-religious meditations on the ethics of genetics and its applications (Bosk 1992)—how genuine were they really? Might they have not taken place if I had been absent and subjects felt no obligation to show just how seriously they took those obligations in which I was most interested? I did not much entertain these doubts at the time of the fieldwork. The data were often too good to question in this way. But now I wonder if I need to reconsider how an attentive audience of one with a tape recorder or stenographer's notebook, taking down every word, might cause a self-conscious subject to play his or her social role "over the top." Because such role performances make the task of the ethnographer so much easier, ethnographers have little incentive for asking these questions in this way. In fact, incentives run the other way, leading researchers to dismiss the possibility of such observer effects. But if I am able to sustain my role performance for the duration of the fieldwork, why is the same not true of those who are observed?

Questions of observer effect aside, it is worth returning to "cover stories" and paying attention to what they do not discuss and what ethnographers avoid discussing up-front. First, for methodological reasons, ethnographers obscure or keep vague their research questions. Next, ethnographers do not discuss what the experience of being observed might be like for subjects. Subjects who are curious or apprehensive about the impact of observation routinely are assured that impacts are benign, that the researcher is just one more "hale fellow well met," who would never, ever, interfere with the ongoing group process. Researchers assume that subjects who wish to avoid observation will find ways to do so. We certainly feel little obligation to spell out a subject's right not to participate. We routinely promise confidentiality and anonymity, but we do not discuss how this promise is easy to make but difficult to fulfill.

I do not mean to imply that ethnographers do not take moral obligations seriously. The literature provides a fairly standardized corpus of ethical questions, spectacular examples of questionable behavior in the past, and a lively debate about our professional responsibilities. For example, to preserve confidentiality, ethnographers have accepted incarceration. This certainly is evidence of serious moral commitment. By the same token, to gather data otherwise unobtainable, ethnographers have conducted covert observations and then worried in their texts about the appropriateness of doing so. Ethnographers have endangered themselves for their subjects; and they have, unwittingly, endangered their subjects in their publications. None of these are topics that a researcher worried about access and entry would choose to mention to a potential but reluctant research subject. All of this suggests nothing less than that the world is a morally complex place. This is not news. What I wish to point out here is something else: our sociological imagination has been dulled by repeatedly grinding it against the same issues. Fieldwork is more morally complex than the constant rehearsal of the same issues suggests. In general, our discussions of rapport, of confidentiality, of the codes of conduct for researchers evade rather than confront the moral complexities of fieldwork. It is this subject to which I now turn.

Ethnography as a Morally Problematic Activity

As a human activity, fieldwork is most peculiar because it contravenes so many of the ordinary rules of everyday social life. It is not just that researchers who do fieldwork watch social life as it unfolds and then report on it, in the process airing much of a group's dirty linen (although we ethnographers do that for certain); it is not just that ethnographers take a group's most cherished notions of itself and show how these are self-serving (although we do that for certain as well); rather, it is how ethnographers do these things that makes fieldwork sometimes feel like such a morally dubious human activity. The key word here is human. Fieldwork is, whatever its difficulties, often redeemed by the fact that it is a human activity. It involves living with and coming to know a group of "strangers." Other research methods are not quite so humanly involving. Of field methods, I feel as others may feel about democracy—it is a terrible method; it is just better (for the kinds of questions that intrigue me) than all the alternatives. This, more than anything else, allows me to engage in the multiple morally dubious behaviors described below.

First, ethnographers trade quite freely on an almost universal misunderstanding between our research subjects and ourselves. For most subjects, the opportunity to be studied is flattering: it feeds or confirms a sense of specialness; it is a vehicle for being lifted out of the ordinary and everyday; and it is even seen by some as a backdoor to an obscure, academic immortality. Because our subjects are flattered by our attention, we are allowed to obtain data that it is not necessarily in our subjects' best interest to reveal. Few of us have ever reported that we inform our subjects of this fact. Rather, because it so often serves our purposes so well, we encourage any misperceptions that yield rich data.

Exactly what makes data rich, what allows data to sustain a "thick description" (Geertz 1973), is hard to specify absent a concrete situation. However, a rule of thumb is easy to provide: rich data subvert official definitions, generally accepted public understandings, and conventional wisdom. Such data tell us what public records and official statistics conceal. Such data are best gathered backstage, behind the yellow tape and the sign limiting access to authorized personnel. Above all, rich data are data that allow the observer the opportunity to interpret social life ironically.

In so doing, we ethnographers betray our subjects twice: first, when we manipulate our relationship with subjects to generate data and then again when we retire to our desks to transform experience to text. This second betrayal is the one my subjects have felt the most keenly. It is the one about which they have complained. Whether it causes them to reevaluate the quasi-friendship we had during the time I was conducting the fieldwork, I do not know (and, in truth, would probably prefer not to know). Both surgeons and genetic counselors felt misrepresented by my attempts to provide what I—but not they—considered an objective description of their occupational world. This sense of betrayal did not center on the accuracy of my description. Both surgeons and genetic counselors agreed that things had happened as I had described them. Their sense of betrayal centered on the contexts within which I placed the description of incidents rather than the incidental description itself.

After reviewing my manuscript for *Forgive and Remember* (1979), the chair of surgery objected to my framing my discussion of mistakes in a sociological rhetoric borrowed from the vocabulary of deviance and social control. He felt, and he let me know that a number of other attendings who had also read the manuscript also felt, that this language was entirely inappropriate:

surgery was too noble a profession for this treatment. He suggested that he, and those other nonspecified colleagues who shared his concern and with whom he had discussed the problem, would prefer a discussion in terms of suboptimal performance rather than mistakes. He and his colleagues felt that all this talk of deviance obscured the background of excellence against which the incidents I described so accurately—and here there was a mixture of flattery and amazement in his tone—came to be thought of as mistakes. I told him that I appreciated his and his colleagues' concerns, that I was grateful for the places in the text where they corrected technical details and misspellings to rescue me from embarrassment, that I was happy to remove an offending phrase here or a too revealing detail there, but that was all. The sociological interpretation was my business, not his. It was the domain where I was the expert. It was his and his colleagues' life but my interpretation. He was not happy. We were both surprised by my assertion of authorial privilege, given the differences in age and rank between us. But, somewhat grudgingly, he yielded—it was my interpretation, after all; and there was still some question in both our minds as to whether it would ever see the light of day.

The same issue of interpretive license arose after my informants read a prepublication version of *All God's Mistakes* (1992). I remember dropping the text off at the office of the genetic counselor who in the text is known as Bill Smith. He received the text with what seemed to be genuine joy—a huge grin followed by a warm hug—at my having completed a much-delayed project. As I waited, Bill, with a new assistant whom I had just met, began to leaf through the text, starting with the table of contents. Joy quickly turned to a mixture of horror, fear, and disapproval. "'A Mop-Up Service, Janitors, Shock Absorbers.'. . . Oh no . . . Bosk, you can't say this," said Bill. The assistant responded, "But why not, you say it every day." Bill told her, "That's different. I say it to you, to the walls of my office, to the conference room. It's one thing for you all to know what I think. It's another to put it out there for everyone to see. How will I work with these people?"

I thought at the time that Bill Smith's reaction encapsulated all that had made him such an interesting subject: an over-the-top, heart-on-his-sleeve, quickly verbalized emotional reaction to an unexpected situation. Such responses were as transient as they were entertaining. I expected Bill to adjust. I was wrong. Late that afternoon when I returned to my office there was a call from the hospital attorney of Nightingale Children's Hospital. She informed me that Bill Smith was very upset and had called her to discuss the possibility of blocking publication. I asked, "On what grounds?" She said that Smith and the others in the work group felt that their identities were not blinded sufficiently. As a result, they felt that the work "held them up to public ridicule and irreparably harmed, their professional reputations." In addition, the lawyer stated, all of my subjects claimed to be unaware that I was doing the research for the purpose of writing a book. Or, alternatively, they claimed (and at this point in the conversation, I was having some difficulty sorting out exactly what was being said, and even with very precise notes am having some difficulty reconstructing it now) that they thought I was studying patients and not the professional staff. Therefore, I had gained these data without their fully informed consent. Finally, they claimed to be worried about patient confidentiality, and, because I had not received formal consent to either observe sessions or interview patients, I could not publish the data.

My first response was pugnacious. I suggested to the attorney that if my subjects wanted to turn an obscure academic treatise into a First Amendment issue, that was fine with me—I could hardly hope to get so much free publicity any other way. The lawyer attempted to soothe me. She told me that that was just the sort of thing she wanted to avoid, that these physicians had thought of me as their friend and now they felt betrayed (a feeling with which she agreed, given her quick skim of the manuscript), and that she was offering her services to broker an amicable settlement. She asked if I could let her know when I would be available over the next few days for a meeting.

After a few phone calls back and forth, we agreed that I was to meet with my former friends and research subjects who were now my current adversaries the next morning. I spent a troubled night. Because the research proposal from which the manuscript grew had been submitted originally as part of a National Institutes of Health "Center" grant, the claim that my subject/ informants had not known that they were the object of my attention was clearly not correct. My institution's institutional review board had approved the actual study; I had a drawerful of consent forms. I felt that all of my former friends' complaints were baseless. Yet, I also understood that the literal truth was not the most critical issue here. The more I thought about it—and try as I might I could not think of anything else—the more anxious I was, even though I knew bruised feelings were a "natural" part of good fieldwork. I had been taught that, in making the latent manifest, the fieldworker made his or her subjects uncomfortable. And I was also taught that this discomfort, which was likened to resistance in psychoanalytic theory, indicated that the ethnographic interpretation had some substance: an account that did not make subjects squirm was suspect, because it showed that the researcher had not penetrated deeply enough into the social world being described. What I had been taught, I was now teaching to my graduate students. Cognitively, I knew what the words meant. I even understood that such beliefs served to protect fieldworkers emotionally by providing a rationale for understanding and then dismissing subjects' negative reactions to our work. However, I had never been brought face-to-face with the consequences of this belief system. It was an educational experience I would have preferred to avoid.

But that was not an option. So, there I was that next morning, sitting across from folks whose social world I long ago shared but who were now strangers—very angry strangers. And really there was more to it than that. As I discussed in *All God's Mistakes* (1992), I was invited by the genetic counselors to study them and their social world. They wanted help as they entered socially uncharted waters. They asked for help and what they felt they got instead was public humiliation. I had always been aware of this as a possible outcome. My fears about this, in fact, slowed the writing of this volume. It was a task I avoided for many years until all the junior colleagues involved in the fieldwork had either been promoted or not. Although I always realized that one consequence of the writing would be to confront some very hurt colleagues, I always assumed that such confrontations would be unplanned, would take place on social occasions, and would be contained by those occasions.

I never expected to confront colleagues in a meeting called specifically so that they could tell me exactly how badly I had wronged them. On the advice of a friend and colleague at the University of Pennsylvania Law School, I brought along two observers. Because there were going to be three of my former colleagues present, my friend thought I ought to have an equal number of allies in the room. This way if there were a dispute later about what we agreed to, it would not simply be a matter of my word against theirs. My observers played no role in the subsequent negotiations, although they did provide comfort and support. Their presence was objected to by my former colleagues, but, at my insistence, they remained.

The meeting began with Bill Smith saying that he wished to read a statement. He needed to read the statement, he said, because he was worried that if he just spoke, he would not be able to control himself. He was so mad at me that he had not really thought he would be able to be in the same room with me—a written statement, he said, would let him say what he wanted to say the way he wanted to say it. Bill began to read in a quavering voice—it was clear that he was close to tears—and he was able to get through half his statement before he threw it on the table, turned to one of his colleagues and said simply, "finish," and left the room sobbing.

The statement, as I recall it, was a model of simple eloquence. Bill asserted that he had not slept since reading the manuscript, that he had always been proud of his work, that my work destroyed everything that he had accomplished, that I had in essence done nothing less than erase twenty years of professional achievements, that all of this was harder for him to take because he had always considered me a friend and because he was going through a difficult time in his life, and that if I had even a shard of decency left, I would not publish this book. He was begging me as one human being to another not to publish this book. The colleague who was reading Bill's words looked up after this closing request and said with simple understatement, "I guess you can tell that Bill is pretty upset. We're all a little put out. But the rest of us will get over it. But you have a problem with Bill."

I said that I could see that. I also said that they all should realize that not publishing was not an option. I went on to point out that no one had yet claimed that the book had any misrepresentation of what I had observed. The colleague assured me that what was disturbing, in part, was the accuracy of the description coupled with interpretations with which they did not agree. I said that I was willing to work with them so that the final version of the book made them all less identifiable. However, I would not negotiate without Bill in the room. The colleague promised me that Bill would be present. (This was promised with an aside, "You remember how emotional Bill can be. We'll make sure he is here.")

A few more meetings and we reached an accord. It was a simple thing: A pseudonym here and there was changed to confuse gender and ethnicity. Some of the identifying details of Nightingale Hospital were misstated. (The hospital attorney asked me to change the bed number. It mattered little to her if I inflated or deflated the figure—either would do, as long as it was inaccurate.) I was asked to change a few rare diseases so patient confidentiality would not be compromised. The genetic counselors were helpful in identifying other rare disorders with the same risk of recurrence, mode of inheritance, and likelihood of prenatal diagnosis. We haggled a bit over some interpretive terms such as "mop-up service." But my line in the sand held firm: if the details were wrong, I would change them; if the details threatened to breach confidentiality and anonymity, I would blur them; if any extraneous remark, an aside in the flow of interaction, was likely to raise hackles unnecessarily, I would remove it; but the interpretation was, rightly or wrongly, for better or worse, mine.

Not surprisingly, this is the stance that has a great deal of legitimacy in an institution such as the modern tertiary care hospital, where professional turf and authority routinely are challenged and defended. That it is built out of a largely illusory distinction, that it is not so easy to disentangle facts from interpretive frameworks, that the authorial privilege, which I claimed rested on an expertise that is easily questioned—none of these issues were raised. Nor was a more troubling issue raised—that the sense of betrayal of the genetic counselors of Nightingale Children's Hospital, similar to that of the surgeons of Pacific Hospital before them, rested on a quite firm basis in reality. I had in some larger sense operated without informed consent. I had violated confidentiality and anonymity. Beyond that, these breaches were both inescapable and reasonably foreseeable. In fact, I believe it is impossible to do hospital-based ethnography without both violating informed consent and without breaking promises made to subjects about confidentiality and anonymity.

There is a trivial sense in which ethnographers cannot help but operate without informed consent. As strangers come and go in the environment, we cannot break up the flow of interaction to tell each newcomer that they have just entered a "research zone," that their words are likely to be recorded, and that their actions may be described and interpreted in a text at a later date. An overly scrupulous approach to informed consent would create disruptions of social life, would be intrusive, would heighten self-consciousness of actors to a high degree, and would be so socially bizarre that it would make fieldwork impossible to complete. But I think that this is something everyone recognizes and that no one expects every person who enters the field to be informed that they have just become an extra in someone else's social drama. However, there is a deeper level at which we breach the spirit of informed consent. We mislead subjects about our intentions and keep them in the dark about reasonable and easily recognized risks, even when our subjects understand (and misunderstand) our role—when they tell us, "I see, you're Malinowski and we are the Trobrianders," or when they inform us of their willingness to be subjects: "Oh yes, how we manage uncertainty, how we handle mistakes, how we define professional service, how we cope with pressure and stress—those are interesting questions. Of course, you can observe." We describe our intent, but we omit a detail. We disclose but only incompletely.

What we leave out is more important than what we choose to reveal. Of all that goes unsaid, the most important element is the hardest to explain, yet at the same time, it is fundamental for understanding the feelings of betrayal that subjects and informants so routinely experience. Subjects, being human, are flattered by our attention. Subjects, especially physicians in bureaucratic organizations, often feel beleaguered by demands from both patients and hospital administration. A common complaint is that dedicated service is unappreciated. A common sentiment is that if only the nature of the pressures on harried doctors were really understood, if only the complexities of the work were truly known, and if only the self-sacrifice were more visible, then physicians would receive more of the public esteem that many in the occupation feel they deserve but currently are denied. It is these negative sentiments and their potential correction—this sense of being chronically misunderstood—that fieldworkers tap into when they seek access to medical settings. Into this situation the ethnographer walks and tells his or her subjects, who feel so misunderstood, what they most want to hear. What the fieldworker promises to describe and explain—the subjects' world from the subjects' point of view—is the story most subjects want desperately to have told. Physicians who know the social science literature, and they are not so numerous as one might hope, know that their wishes here may outrun reality. They may intuit that being understood is more than they can hope for, but a number of powerful forces countervail: the support for inquiry in academic medical centers and the lack of alternatives for having their stories told are two of the most important.

There would be nothing wrong with this if all or most of what we were interested in was the "world from the actors' point of view." But that is not the case, regardless of our disclaimers to the contrary. All good fieldwork must describe the "world from the actors' point of view," must record accurately what Geertz (1973) calls "the said" of social life, but this is the starting point—a necessary but not a sufficient element in producing adequate ethnography. Ethnographers do not inform subjects that the world from their point of view is the starting point for our interpretive activities. It is through these interpretations that subjects feel the sense of betrayal at ethnographic portraits of their social world. And this is not surprising because what is most unsettling to subjects about ethnographic interpretations is built into the way social scientists are socialized to think about the world.

The most characteristic ways a social scientist learns to think are organized to disabuse any group of its own notions of its "specialness." Social science is a generalizing activity. One implication of this is that when group members claim special qualities, sensitivities, skills, or privileges, ethnographers dutifully record these sentiments. We take the sacred beliefs of a group about itself seriously but not literally; and social scientists do more. We point out how such sentiments are shared by other groups and are manipulated by those groups for their own advantage; we show how altruistic beliefs cloak self-interest. In short, what we do is take a group's sense of its specialness and inspect it; and while inspecting it, we show how ordinary, common-place, and self-serving it really is. Few groups are grateful for this.

What in all of this violates the spirit of informed consent? At the simplest level, I suppose it is no more complicated than this. Experienced ethnographers know that nothing is so prized in the social science literature as the counterintuitive finding, that no voice is so cultivated as the ironic, and that no spirit characterizes work so much as a debunking one. Yet we certainly do not warn our subjects of this. One might say that this is trivial—there is risk in all of this, but the harm is negligible. I am not so sure. I lost my certitude in the harmlessness of my methods and of my ways of describing them to my subjects on the morning Bill Smith tossed his written statement on the table and fled the room crying.

One might argue that, even if the risks of irony were explained, subjects would not be able to understand them; they would consent anyway and still feel betrayed in the end. After all, we social scientists expect to see the world from the subject's point of view, but we have the benefit of extensive professional training. How can we expect our subjects to intuit our objectives, to see the world clearly from our point of view? These are not arguments that are given much credence when physicians use them as an excuse for failing to provide patients the data necessary for informed consent. They possess no more credence when given by social scientists as a justification for less than full disclosure. The simple fact is that we do not try to explain this aspect of our work to our subjects, and we feel no obligation to try for this level of consent. The simplest explanation is that such disclosure is difficult; it does indeed impede our ability to gather our data and do our work. If this is the case, then these difficulties need to be confronted. Pretending that they do not exist is not an adequate response for the social scientist or any other researcher.

But there is another reason we do not feel duty-bound to disclose to subjects that ultimately they will feel betrayed by our ethnographic reports. The act of betrayal occurs after we have left the field. It occurs when we are no longer engaged with our subjects and when we no longer need their cooperation. Moreover, few of us are ever confronted by the egos our work bruises, the souls it lacerates, or the communal relationships it roils. This aspect of our work is not something we see, something we have to live with. Very few sociological ethnographers ever return to the same site for further explorations.

Nor is this the only way our consent procedures are flawed. Our disclosures about confidentiality and anonymity are likewise inadequate. Here, too, the problem lies more with what we do not say than with what we do. We routinely promise confidentiality and anonymity. Even when subjects have requested to be clearly identified or have had no objections to being identified, I have resisted. In part, I resist because confidentiality serves separate ends of my own. However much they protect subjects, confidentiality and anonymity are important rhetorical devices for ethnographic reportage. They transform the specific into the general. This surgical ward becomes the world of surgery. This blighted urban neighborhood becomes every urban neighborhood. Without confidentiality and anonymity, arguments about this transformation and about the representativeness that it effortlessly provides would be even more tedious and never-ending than they already are.

There is an irony, though, in our sincere promise of confidentiality and anonymity and in our clumsy efforts to achieve it. We succeed where it matters least and fail where it matters most. For those far from the scene, our pseudonyms effectively disguise the location of our investigations and the identity of our subjects. But then for these readers little would matter if we named actual names, because our subjects rarely are known outside local circles. But none of this is true in the actual community where the research was done. Here no attempt to disguise is ever wholly adequate. One could argue that this is a reason for multiple-site case studies. However, this solution compounds the problem rather than solves it. Subjects, and the colleagues of subjects, can read the ethnographer's writings, and this reading poses a real, if largely unacknowledged, risk to the research from the subject's point of view.

The risk is the one that Bill Smith recognized immediately, even if too late, when he first skimmed the text of *All God's Mistakes:* I said those things about my colleagues, but I didn't realize that they would see them. Now that they will, how can I continue to work with them? Not only was Smith's complaint justified, but I also should have anticipated it on the basis of my past experience. In *Forgive and Remember,* all of my attempts to conceal the identity of individuals and the organization failed most spectacularly at Pacific Hospital. To this day, the place where *Forgive and Remember* moves most briskly off the shelves is the Pacific University bookstore. The hospital staff there at all levels and from all departments read the book as a *roman à clef.* And this remains so despite the fact that with the passage of time, few of my original subjects are still at Pacific. Yet the readers on the Pacific payroll have no trouble figuring out who is who. For years, informants have told me that these successful decodings always provide a secret, guilty pleasure to readers: "Ah ha, so he really thought that." "That's just like him to behave that poorly." "Boy, I'm glad I don't have to deal directly with that son of a bitch." Having failed so spectacularly at providing confidentiality and anonymity once before at the place where it was most necessary, I should have anticipated Bill Smith's objection.

The issue is deeper than a single unkept promise. The decoding of the text by locals has consequences; as Schutz (1962) was so fond of saying, it "gears into the world." Consider the data of most interest to members of the local institution: the airing of dirty laundry in public and statements about colleagues' behaviors made behind their back in the heat of a private moment. Such statements are like letters written in anger; but unlike such letters, they have been sent, received, and digested. Such statements also are similar to angry remarks directed to another in public. But unlike public remarks, they do not provide the opportunity to respond to a colleague's hurt feelings. Social life provides wiggle room; texts on social life do not. The very fact that such criticisms are made behind closed doors is an indicator that those making them did not want them displayed before an audience. When I am an audience of one for such "emotional flooding out," I use every means I know to keep the affect flowing. This means that the revelations that I make public often go further than subjects intended. Certainly, the text always contains more than subjects would reveal if I routinely said at such moments, "Are you sure you want to go there? Remember, I'm taking notes. Someday this all might appear in a book that your colleagues will be able to read."

There is, then, a very real risk that derives from the utter impossibility of maintaining confidentiality and anonymity at a local level. The atmosphere of naive trust that makes work possible is placed in jeopardy. The world becomes a less happy place. It is hard to know how to warn of these risks, because they share so little with the ordinary risks of social life. We frank postmoderns at the beginning of the twenty-first century place a high value on candor. Our subjects likely are to believe mistakenly that they are the kind of people who would never say anything in private that they would not say in public. They may even pride themselves on this self-deception to their later chagrin. All of this serves to illustrate that, as Goffman (1961) so epigrammatically and enigmatically put it in another context, "Life may not be much of a gamble, but interaction is." And Goffman forgot to add, "Interaction is a gamble against much longer odds when there is an ethnographer present."

Conclusion: Ethnographer-Ethicist Beware

Philosophers who advocate a more narrative, more deeply contextualized, more socially situated bioethics often point to the ethnographies of medical sociologists as examples of the kind of work they have in mind (Hoffmaster 1992). The implication is that if only ethicists either used or did more of this sort of work, if they only provided a "thicker description," then much of the ambiguity and uncertainty embedded in principlist approaches to bioethics would disappear.

This essay has been an oblique plea for philosophers to look elsewhere for help. The rationales offered have been largely pragmatic or emotional/moral. Ethnography invariably involves deception. Subjects misread the ethnographer's interest in their world, and ethnographers take no pains to correct these misreadings. Subjects do not understand that ethnographers debunk what Becker (1968) called "conventional sentimentality," the commonly accepted social versions of virtue and vice; that ethnographers write in an arch, ironic voice; that the objective of ethnographic writing often is to "debunk"; and that this debunking is accomplished by showing how altruistic statements hide self-interested motives. When subjects read what is written about them, they often feel betrayal. Beyond that, the doing of ethnography often rests on promises of confidentiality and anonymity that are invariably broken and, if not broken, at the very least are made without any confidence in or control over whether they will be kept.

These deceptions and broken promises ethnographers are willing to accept. As researchers, ethnographers are willing to apply a utilitarian calculus. The knowledge gained is worth the harm inflicted (at least as far as the researcher is concerned). And, if truth be told, these deceptions and broken promises are not usually a problem. The typical sociological ethnography focuses on those low in status hierarchies, those who command little respect, and those who are demonized by respectable society. Debunking in these circumstances means showing that those who might otherwise be thought of as moral monsters are really rational and honorable creatures, living within the rules of their subcultures. So, for such subjects, ethnography actually elevates their moral status. Because few of these subjects read our accounts, the potential for harm is minimal. However, all this changes when ethnogra-

phers study high-status groups. Debunking in this situation involves the ethnographer showing that those with noble social position are more base than
commonly realized. Here, subjects are highly literate, and ethnographers
can do harm in local settings where their work, if read, can destroy mutual
trust. Unfortunately, this is a problem that is easier to identify than to remedy. Even so, as far as ethnographers are concerned, there is no other way to
go about the research. If what the ethnographer writes is truthful—leaving
to one side, for the moment, the complexities involved in making such an
assessment—this is a defense all its own. If the shoe pinches, if the facts are
inconvenient, that is what Weber (Gerth and Mills 1956) so long ago told us
that science as a vocation was about.

But even if they satisfy social scientists, for ethicists these justifications
are not wholly adequate. If one wishes to "do" ethics, there is an expectation
that one will be above reproach. The manipulations, deceptions, evasions,
and silences, without which it is impossible to gather data, make it hard
for any ethnographer—no matter how pure his or her motivation, no matter how scrupulous his or her conduct—to be above reproach. In short, to
produce a more narrative ethics, to introduce ethnographic methods into
bioethics, may force the ethicist to act in ways that give lie to the claim, "I
am an ethicist."

If ethicist were a role like ethnographer, that is to say, if the ethicist did
research in one place and taught in another, then perhaps the moral failings
embedded in the research process would not be of much moment. Alternatively, if ethicist were one of those roles where there was no expectation of a
relationship between knowing and doing, then the betrayals and deceptions
of the researcher would not count for much. But matters are not so simple.
For ethicists, there is a role-based incompatibility between the doing of ethics and the doing of ethnography.

Since Simmel (Levine 1970), ethnographers often have claimed their
unique purchase on social life is made possible because they are "strangers"
to the scenes they explore. As such, they possess a paradoxical combination
of nearness and distance, remoteness and intimacy. The world at hand, to
lapse for a moment into phenomenological jargon, is both accessible and
puzzling. Of course, by the end of an intensive fieldwork experience, the
ethnographer is no longer a stranger. The world at hand is now familiar; its
original mysteries are now nothing more than a set of everyday routines,
contingent accomplishments, and repeated occurrences. More than anything else, it is this loss of stranger status for the fieldworker and of phenom-

enological puzzlement for the social world that explains the fact that sociological fieldworkers so often flit from site to site or topic to topic rather than
continually try to mine the same settings. Gathering data as an ethnographer
requires a certain skill at playing dumb; any reputation, however minimal,
at being an expert or insider undermines the charade of social stupidity and
thereby makes the research task that much more difficult. Beyond that, in
solving the mysteries of any particular social world, the researcher develops
relationships, makes friends, and builds obligations. This is so even though
the fieldworker is a transient in the studied social world with no role to play
once the research project is completed. The feelings that publication evokes
among subjects then make it difficult to sustain those relationships, retain
those friendships, and honor those obligations.

Unlike ethnographers, bioethicists are usually insiders in hospitals. As
hospital employees, they sit on ethics committees, consult on difficult cases,
teach medical students and residents, and provide a visible presence for ethics. In all this work, they, too, develop relationships, make friends, build
obligations, and have a political stake in the organization. Hospital-based
ethicists work in an environment in which strong norms of confidentiality
exist. If bioethicists were to do ethnography, or even provide examples from
their clinical experience of a more narrative version of ethics, they would
need to trade on those relationships, betray some of those friendships, ignore some of those obligations, and tread, however lightly, on those norms of
confidentiality. For bioethicists, the work of "displaying the data" might very
well involve airing some dirty organizational linen that could transform insiders in hospitals to outsiders. This, then, may compromise the bioethicist's
effectiveness as a front-line worker, as a committee member, as a consultant,
as a teacher, and as a visible symbol of ethics.

Put most simply, if bioethicists themselves heed the call to produce a
more contextual, a more narrative ethics, they may undercut their effectiveness in their other organizational roles. Studying some things one way makes
it impossible to do other things in other ways. To that problem, we may add
another. Full participation, a stake in outcomes, makes it difficult to achieve
the distance that is part of what makes ethnographic interpretation possible.
Partisan accounts often are detailed and very convincing, serve a purpose,
and provide a unique window into a social world. They are many things; but
one thing they are not is ethnography.

There is, of course, a difference between doing and using, creating and
appreciating, making and applying. A more contextual bioethics does not re-

quire that bioethicists become ethnographers. But ethnography, as currently practiced by ethnographers, is not likely to produce accounts all that useful to bioethicists. For that to be so, ethnographers would need to be trained to take the normative as seriously as they take the empirical, to see the normative as something more substantial than a reflection of material interests and the cultural values associated with them. There is very little in social science theory or training that allows for this now. Nor are current trends any reason to feel sanguine about the future. Further, if ethnographers were to make the ethical dilemmas of the bedside the subject of their inquiries, then the everyday work of bioethicists would become the observational basis of their interpretive activities. This places bioethics in context to be sure; but it does so without necessarily producing an account of how the work of ethics is done that would be useful to bioethicists. After all, such accounts would be marked by that ironic and debunking tone that invariably creates tensions between ethnographers and their subjects.

References

Anspach, Renee R. 1993. *Deciding Who Lives: Fateful Choices in the Intensive-Care Nursery.* Berkeley: University of California Press.

Becker, Howard. 1968. Whose Side Are We On? *Social Problems* 14:239–247.

Bluebond-Langner, Myra. 1978. *The Private Worlds of Dying Children.* Princeton, NJ: Princeton University Press.

Bosk, Charles L. 1979. *Forgive and Remember: Managing Medical Failure.* Chicago: University of Chicago Press.

———. 1992. *All God's Mistakes: Genetic Counseling in a Pediatric Hospital.* Chicago: University of Chicago Press.

Edin, Kathryn, and Laura Lein. 1997. *Making Ends Meet: How Single Mothers Survive Welfare and Low-Wage Work.* New York: Russell Sage Foundation.

Geertz, Clifford. 1973. *The Interpretation of Cultures.* New York: Basic Books.

Gerth, Hans, and C. W. Mills. 1956. *From Max Weber.* Glencoe, IL, and New York: Free Press.

Goffman, Erving. 1961. *Interaction Ritual.* New York: Pantheon.

Hoffmaster, Barry. 1992. Can Ethnography Save the Life of Medical Ethics? *Social Science and Medicine* 35:1421–1431.

Klockars, Carl. 1974. *The Professional Fence.* New York: Free Press.

Levine, Donald. 1971. *Georg Simmel: On Individuality and Social Forms.* Chicago: University of Chicago Press.

Park, Robert, and Ernest Burgess. [1922] 1967. *The City.* Chicago: University of Chicago Press.

Sanchez-Jankowski, Martin. 1991. *Islands in the Street: Gangs and American Urban Society.* Berkeley: University of California Press.

Schutz, Alfred. 1962. *The Collected Papers*, Vol. 1. The Hague: Martinus Nijhoff.

Van Maanen, John. 1988. *Tales of the Field: On Writing Ethnography*. Chicago: University of Chicago Press.

Whyte, William Foote. 1955. *Street Corner Society*. Chicago: University of Chicago Press.

Zussman, Robert. 1992. *Intensive Care: Medical Ethics and the Medical Profession*. Chicago: University of Chicago Press.

3

THE ETHICS OF ETHNOGRAPHY

SURGEONS REVISITED

NINE

The Field-Worker and the Surgeon

All fieldwork done by a single field-worker invites the question, Why should we believe it? It would be nice to be able to claim that I was a totally impartial observer whose characteristic ways of looking at the world allow an almost perfect mirroring of some objective reality. However, as the fieldwork experience made clear to me, I am not without my biases. I would like to pretend that this was not so for any number of reasons, but the observer role in some sense trained me to see these biases in a heightened way. As I reflect on the experience of eighteen months of participant observation in a teaching hospital, and on the dilemmas of the observer role, I feel a sense of respect for data-collecting procedures which allow the researcher to keep the sensuous world at a distance, and which thereby allow him to avoid the self-exposure, self-reflection, and self-doubt endemic to field-workers. In the field, the everyday life of his subjects overwhelms the researcher, threatens to obliterate his sense of self, and forces a reconsideration of deeply held personal and intellectual beliefs. It would be of little point, then, for me to pretend in the face of such a powerful experience that I was merely a coding machine which transcribed the events of everyday life first into field material and then into the sociological and literary order of the preceding pages. In this chapter, I would like to describe the field experience itself and the analysis of the data. This chapter should show the reader how I identified

Chapter 9 was originally published as Charles L. Bosk, "The Field-Worker and the Surgeon," in *Forgive and Remember: Managing Medical Failure.* (Chicago: University of Chicago Press, 1979), 193–213.

and controlled for my own biases and should allow him to control for them independently of me.

In the Field

How did I begin? The first thing I did was to approach an attending I had met at a party, explain my proposed study, and ask for his cooperation. The attending expressed enthusiasm for the project, but refused his cooperation. He claimed that if I wanted to really be trusted, I would need the housestaff's acceptance. He expressed his fear that his sponsorship would be a "kiss of death": housestaff would view me as his spy and never talk freely with me. If I wanted my project to succeed, he advised, I needed to be seen as my own person. So rather than somehow magically start the research, he gave me the names of a number of residents and the hospital's central page number. What I learned during this interview was that there was no instant access for the field-worker. Not sure if I was receiving aid or a run-around from my initial contact, I called the first name on his list, the chief resident. We met for coffee and I explained my plans. The resident approved my being an observer on his service, but claimed he would have to check with both attendings. The chairman of my department provided a letter of introduction to the chairman of the Department of Surgery. Gaining my initial entrée was a multi-staged diplomatic problem. Each interaction was a test, and access was the result of continual testing and retesting. Entrée was not something negotiated once and then over and done with. I was always entering new scenes and situations involving different combinations of people. Fortunately, of course, I could rely on what I had learned in previous encounters and the repertoire of roles that I had developed and that others developed for me. The important thing that field-workers must keep in mind is that entrée is not a single event but a continuous process.

Access—being allowed in the scene—is one thing, but approval and trust of field subjects is quite another. Just like access, cooperation cannot be ordered by fiat, but is rather earned again and again, when the field-worker shows that he or she is trustworthy and reliable. Much is made in fieldwork accounts of the "cover story" which the observer uses to explain his presence in the setting as a first and essential step in gaining trust. My cover story was very simple. I explained that I was doing a dissertation on the way surgeons learned to recognize and control error. The surgeons were, as a rule, remarkably uncurious about my research. None ever questioned the legitimacy of my research question or the nature of my methods during our initial meetings. Few even requested that I account for my presence. I was not asked for my cover story very often and, when asked for the story, I was not required to elaborate on it. In some sense, my access was secured by sponsorship of housestaff trusted by all. Once my access was established, my cover story was superfluous and served as a gloss during introductions. In the everyday course of things, my housestaff sponsor was more important to my access than any cover story I used.

Trust was gained neither during initial introductions nor by the artful manipulation of a cover story, but through my performance in roles I assumed and was assigned by housestaff and attendings. Housestaff assigned me a number of roles. Most generally, I was an "extra pair of hands," and a "gofer." During the time of my fieldwork, I became very proficient at opening packages of bandages, retrieving charts, and fetching items from the supply room. Through these tasks, I expressed some solidarity with whatever group I was observing and gave something, however inconsequential, in exchange for "observing rights." Second, I was an "emissary from the outside world." My round of life was less circumscribed than a houseofficer's: I read and watched more news, saw more movies, and participated more fully in university life outside the hospital. In some sense, I provided housestaff contact with a world they felt cut off from. During Watergate, I always brought a number of papers into the hospital. How or why this became my task I do not know. Often I purchased these papers at the hospital gift stand, a place interns and residents certainly had access to. Their general reluctance to pick such papers up is not so much a mark of their frugality as a symbolic statement about their relation to the world outside Pacific Hospital. I later learned that housestaff attach a magical property to newspapers, books, and magazines. If they bring them in to work they see this as jinxing themselves and condemning the group to an impossibly busy day. It is, however, permissible for outsiders to bring such taboo items to them. My passing remarks about movies, current events, the weather—all were taken as an indication of what educated people on the outside were thinking. Third, I was a "fellow-sufferer." As a graduate student not released from training, I was perceived as occupying a position analagous to the houseofficer's. My own career problems and expectations were topics that houseofficers initiated much conversation about. They constantly compared and contrasted our different experiences. During such exchanges, houseofficers constantly emphasized the indignity of their roles and often suggested that their present burdens justified their future rewards. From me, they sought to learn about the generalized indignities of the subordinate role in sociological training. I regaled them with my wildest recollections of coding data and proofreading galleys.

Fourth, I was a convenient "sounding board." I was surprised at the degree that informants sought me out to relate stories of practice that they disagreed with. Feelings that were not shared in the group, discontents, uncertainties were taken to me. I knew that observers were often sought by organizational malcontents; what surprised me was that all my informants were at one time or another malcontents. Such a label was not a stable organizational identity as much as a fleeting reaction to behavior, which for one reason or another offended the houseofficer's sensibilities. Disfiguring palliative operations, patient discomfort, and the openness of communications among the ranks were the most common complaints. As a "sounding board," I was implicitly asked to play a quasi-therapeutic role: to listen without judging and to understand. The fact that I was asked to play this role so often by so many speaks both to their understanding of what an observer does and to the deep feelings that physicians repress as a matter of course. As a rule, we, as medical sociologists, have not concentrated enough on how fragile physician defenses are, what events disturb them, and how primal the existential material they are dealing with is. Birth, life, death are not questions that one works through definitively. We need to pay more attention to the provisional nature of the resolution physicians make to the conflicts such subjects present. My own graduate students in the field now report that their informants ask them to play this quasi-therapeutic role, also. Like me, they find it both disturbing and flattering. The fact that our subjects choose to use us in this way suggests both that we need to learn methods for containing and managing these encounters, and also that we cannot define the field-worker role totally in instrumental terms. We come to have identities for our subjects quite independent of the ones we promote for ourselves. Ironically, it is often these identities that yield the greatest amount of data.

Fifth, houseofficers viewed me as a "referee" in conflicts among themselves over patient management, quarrels over the equity of the division of labor, and disputes about whether or not patients understood what was happening. In the midst of such disagreements, one houseofficer would turn to me and ask: "Well, what do you think? Which of us is right?" These were not comfortable situations for me when I could hide behind the observer role. A judgment was demanded as the price for my continued presence. Moreover, any judgment was certain to alienate one of my informants. I developed tactics for throwing the question back to the disputants or for pointing out the merits of either side, or making a joke of the entire dispute. Over time, I tried in vain to teach my subjects that such conflict resolution was not a proper part of my role. Nevertheless, being asked to referee disputes was a recurrent and always problematic task and not one that I ever felt totally comfortable with. As I felt more accepted, I was somewhat better able to put questions off. But in the beginning, I was stiff, uncomfortable, and always mindful of my relationships with each party. As a referee, I was able to elicit good material when I was able to turn the dispute into an occasion for discussing different attitudes and beliefs toward medical practice. Unfortunately, I was not always levelheaded enough to accomplish this because I felt so put-on-the-spot by such confrontations.

Sixth, I was the group "historian." Because of the way house-staff rotate through the various services, it was not unusual for me to have been on either the Able or the Baker Service longer than any particular houseofficer. When this occurred, I was expected to know something of the history of the different patients on the service. I was expected to keep track of attendings' remarks and verify them for absent group members. The role of group historian served me well, since it forced housestaff to depend on me for information that they needed. This created a greater sense of mutual obligation between housestaff and myself and to the degree that the information I supplied was reliable, I established my credibility. Also, I was a short-run as well as long-run historian. I would often ask housestaff about action that I could not watch but was interested in. (Much work is done individually, and on any given day I saw only a portion of possible action.) On more than one occasion, my questioning reminded houseofficers of a task that had until then slipped their minds. My unwitting reminders saved them from oversights which would have gotten them into trouble. The fact that such incidents occurred further indebted housestaff to me and heightened my legitimacy. A field-worker pays a price for this kind of legitimacy, though. The historian role itself presents some of the most common moral dilemmas that a field-worker faces. Each time I gave such a reminder to a houseofficer, I changed what would have otherwise happened without this intervention. Lab tests, consultations with other physicians, and conferences with patients and their families—all these were on occasion events that took place because I reminded houseofficers of them. By jogging the memory of houseofficers in this way, I made it impossible for myself to observe what happens when these events fail to occur. On these occasions, I did not intend to alter the natural course of events; but it did happen that I unwittingly created an occasional participant-observer effect.

Despite the fact that it was not my intention in these instances to change the action I was studying, one can see very clearly that errors of omission present the observer with a moral dilemma. If one does remind a houseofficer, one disturbs by that act the very relationships one is attempting to study. However, if one does not remind the houseofficer—and yet knows he has overlooked something—it is possible that a patient's care will be compromised. On most cases when I asked if something had been done, I did so because as a sociologist I was particularly interested in seeing or hearing a report of that specific action, and usually because I was unaware of whether it had occurred or not—I was trying to orient myself. If the houseofficer had forgotten about the task I was asking about, if it had completely slipped his mind, then that fact told me something about the difference between a sociological perspective and a surgical one; and I learned something more about the structure of the surgeon's life-world. There was one category of event, however—conferences with patients and families—that I asked about more than others. Here I was often conscious of my participation in the scene, but thought that some patients (exactly which patients these were and why I reacted to them the way I did is a complex matter that I do not understand) deserved fuller explanations than they often got from the surgeons. A question that I cannot answer is, Did the surgeons see my role as a sociologist such that they presumed that I was interested in such group phenomena, and did they come to rely on me to remind them of their diffuse obligations to patients and their families? Is this the major role they assigned me in the group? If it was, who was responsible for making sure that this team responsibility was filled when there was no sociologist present? Whatever the answers to these questions, a rule of thumb I applied was to keep my reminders as few as possible. This was a rule I occasionally broke because of my feelings for a patient and his/her family. I must also confess to one other category of event on which I routinely broke my own rule. As a group historian, I occasionally asked questions that served as reminders to subjects that I felt were hostile and/or skeptical of my sociological enterprise to establish that I belonged in the field; that I was concerned, aware and helpful; and that I was a legitimate member of the group. The fact is I occasionally used my questions to demonstrate the ways the group needed me. (One could also argue at the same time I was proving to myself that I served some useful purpose in the group.)

If errors of omission present observers with one type of moral dilemma, errors of commission present him with another. In the case where the fieldworker knows that some harm has been done to a patient through physician or nursing error, does the observer have any direct, ethical obligations to the patient and his/her family? That is, should the field-worker either inform the patient or find some alternative means of making public the error? I chose not to do this for a variety of reasons. As a pragmatic matter, being a patient-advocate would have made the kind of fieldwork I wanted to do impossible. Moreover, I felt a responsibility to other medical sociologists who wished to undertake field projects in the future. I was aware that my conduct could either make the way more or less difficult for those who followed me. While some participant-observer effects seem acceptable to me, others, those that contravene the basic operating norms of a group, are not acceptable. These larger effects not only distort the phenomenon under study, they make it impossible for later field-workers to gain access to and legitimacy within medical settings. Most important, I felt I could discharge my ethical obligations to patients more effectively by describing the general categorization and management of error rather than tilting at windmills in one or two select cases. On the face of it, this kind of advocacy would not seem to be much of a problem; in fact, it is hard to imagine a field-worker, insistent on imposing his definitions of justice on a scene, completing his work. However, this fact is not as significant as the importance of recognizing the strong feelings that observing in a hospital evokes, and restraining the "rescuer" impulses that witnessing so much pain, suffering, and death provokes. Whatever roles houseofficers cast me in or I assumed, the major irony of the field-worker role was always apparent: on the one hand, I was intimately involved in all aspects of the everyday life of a group; and on the other hand, I was constrained by the nature of my task to exert as little social influence in that group as possible. So, my sensitivity to the group's actions and their consequences was heightened at the same time that my theoretic commitments restrained me from even raising the group's consciousness about the effects of its own actions.

I had less intimate contact with attendings than with housestaff, and assumed and was assigned a narrower range of roles. Most commonly, I was seen as any other "medical student." Attendings assimilated me to the group by treating me like any other member of the group. They had me look down proctoscopy tubes, rake abdomens feeling for a mass, and learn to hold retractors properly. Their treatment of me helped strengthen my ties to houseofficers, who saw that not only was I not in league with attendings, but that, like them, I was the occasional butt of an attending's sense of humor. By the same token, my own willingness to take part this way in group life served notice to attendings that I was willing to do what was necessary to complete my project. When attendings viewed me as a medical student, they often tried to teach me concise medical lessons. Whatever problems of identification and rapport I might have had, it is interesting to note that attendings had some of their own. Toward the end of my fieldwork, two attendings approached me, told me that I must be interested in medicine to have spent so much time at Pacific, and then informed me that if I wanted to go to medical school, they would help me in any way they could. I took their offer as an indication that perhaps I had been in the field long enough.

The incident above is related to another role attendings cast me in—their "advisee." Attendings offered two types of advice. First, there was "scientific" advice. Here attendings would address themselves to the design of my study. They wanted to know about my control groups, my measurement instruments, my hypotheses, and all similar paraphernalia from the type of research they engaged in. When I would explain that my model for research was somewhat different than theirs, they were skeptical but generally tolerant. After all, I was the sociology department's problem, and not theirs. Second, attendings offered "interpretive advice." When we were alone, they would often explain why they acted in certain situations the way they did, what they felt to be the burdens of their authority, what the major problems doing surgery in a major medical center were, what the personal strengths and weaknesses of their colleagues were, and so on. Like houseofficers (although the opportunity arose less frequently), attendings unloaded themselves on me. It is worth noting here that I was ten years younger than the youngest attending, so the fact that they used me as a "sounding board" points to ways in which the surgeon's role remains disturbing even to those who have practiced it all of their adult lives.

In addition, attendings used me often as a "clown" to diffuse tensions in the group. When things were going poorly, attendings on occasion would question me like any other member of the group and then poke fun at my fumbling and ignorance. Sitting around the doctors' lounge, the rigors of academic life would be compared unfavorably with those of surgery; and my manly virtues would be impugned. It was not always as a clown that attendings used me to ease tensions. Just as with housestaff, I was asked to referee conflict. My study was used by them to deflect conversations from their course. So that often when faced with troublesome questions from nurses or other physicians, they would give a noncommittal response and then ask me to explain my study. They would ply me with questions until they were sure the conversation could safely resume. These three roles were not assumed with equal frequency nor were all assumed from the first day of fieldwork.

From the beginning and most generally, I was assimilated as a medical student. Then I was used as a "diffuser of tensions," If I passed the test implied in this role, I became an occasional confidant of the attending. With one attending who was not greatly invested in clinical issues, I was never other than a quasi-medical student. With the others, I played all three roles, albeit with varying frequency and intensity.

So far in this description I have concentrated on the various roles I played in the field setting. The rationale for this is simple. In the analysis of our fieldwork data, we concentrate on the role relations among participants in the scene we choose to study. Yet we often pay comparatively less attention to our own role relations with the subjects who make our knowledge of the setting and of the action possible. Since in fieldwork these relationships are our major methodological tool, they require serious discussion. How we manage these relationships determines the depth, validity, and reliability of the data we collect and the inferences we draw from it. We need devices that ensure control of our like and dislike of various participants, the weighting that we give incidents, and the ways our own everyday roles impinge on and create strains with the field-worker role. The problem of objective description and analysis is in itself formidable even if one were only observing a television program, for example. In fieldwork, the problem is made more complex because of the deep relationships and attachments one builds over time to one's subjects. As Charles Lidz (1977) has correctly pointed out, the right and privilege of being an observer is a gift presented to the researcher by his host and subjects. So the observer has, in addition to whatever the other problems that becloud his structured role-relations with his subjects, the very special problems that attend the giving and receiving of gifts. I would agree with Lidz that the recognition and proper understanding of the gift relationship serves as both a convenient theoretical framework for understanding the peculiar dilemmas of the field-worker and at the same time a formidable restraint on bias in observation and interpretation.

First, what are the special features of the gift relationship? As Mauss (1967) pointed out in his classic statement, the giver and the recipient of a gift are involved in an interactional sequence that involves giving, receiving, and reciprocating. Even more important, involvement in a gift cycle creates a solidarity among participants and signifies that they have obligations toward each other that extend into the future. The fact that the field-worker is both the receiver of a gift and a guest means that he has a diffuse sense of obligation to his host-giver-subject. Field-workers have long recognized their indebtedness to their subjects. In fact, as one reads accounts of fieldwork itself one senses that this burden is truly "the magnifcient obsession" of those who employ this research method. While not explicitly analyzing the observer role as a gift relationship, field-workers worry, in their writings, over fulfilling their obligations to their subjects, over balancing personal debts to individuals against universal debts to the discipline of sociology, and over discharging obligations to subjects that extend beyond the life of any particular piece of research. In addition, there is the field-worker's typical ethical dilemma: what if the data I gather are potentially harmful to my subjects? What if the facts themselves betray those to whom I have become so attached over so many months? Others have spoken of the "tyranny of the gift" in different contexts, but it is clear that the gift of access, of witnessing social life as it is lived in someone else's environment, exercises a tyranny of its own. This tyranny has as its most distinctive features three significant elements: (1) the danger of overrapport, so thoroughly merging with the subject's point of view that one cannot achieve the critical distance necessary for analysis; (2) the danger of overindebtedness, so thoroughly feeling a sense of diffuse obligation that one can no longer assess what one does and does not properly owe his subjects; and (3) the danger of overgeneralization, so thoroughly idealizing one's subjects that one sees their behavior as overly representative of all persons in a class.

I was protected from overrapport and overindebtedness in part by the very structure of hospital life. Unlike field-workers who spend years with an unchanging population, my subjects rotated through the surgical services fairly rapidly. Some stayed for as little as a month; none stayed over three months. There were housestaff I liked very much; housestaff I detested; and others I barely got to know, Whatever the case, there was an unending parade of housestaff. The mere fact that I was observing so many people in rapid succession prevented overrapport with any one subject. There was, of course, the danger that I would identify with the structural position of being a houseofficer, even if I avoided strong attachments to specific individuals. After all, I was a twenty-four-year-old graduate student, subordinate to a dissertation committee, and struggling to achieve autonomy within my own profession. Surely there was a clear and ever-present danger that, being a subordinate myself, I would overidentify with the subordinate and his problems. Overrapport with housestaff was avoided by two features of my everyday life. First, my wife, Marjorie Waxman, was supervising child-care workers in a psychiatric hospital at the time of this research. My conversations with her made me sensitive to the problems of the superordinate, especially the difficulty of balancing the needs of patient care with, the needs of subordinates to develop their own skills and judgments through their own mistakes. Second, my major field-supervisor constantly pointed out to me instances when I seemed to take subordinate complaints too much to heart and urged me to see beyond the specific perturbations in housestaff-attending relations to see what are generic problems in superordinate-subordinate relations. Of course, I also had to guard against the opposite problem, overidentification with attendings. After all, did they not have, to an exaggerated degree, the autonomy I was working so hard to obtain? Here, I was' protected from overrapport by a number of factors. First, my relations with attendings were not as regular, intense, or relaxed as those with housestaff. Second, several of my own friends in medical training served as constant reminders of the subordinate's problem. Third, there is a general resistance in sociology to sympathize with the perspective of authority. Authors such as Becker (1970) constantly remind us whose side we should be on.

My resolution to the problem of overindebtedness was somewhat different than the resolution to overrapport, and unfolded over time in two quite separate phases. A moderately sensitive observer of life in the surgery wards of a hospital will be flooded with feelings of helplessness. These feelings themselves have two distinct components. First, witnessing so much pain and suffering, the field-worker wants to roll up his sleeves and do something, anything. At the same time, seeing death as an everyday event makes one guilty and overly aware of one's own good fortune. As a field-worker, I was often made uncomfortable by what I saw. I felt I had stumbled into incredibly intimate and significant slices of patients' and doctors' lives. Much like any person who sees more than he would like of a friend's life, I felt guilty about some of the knowledge I had gained, worried over what the boundary between privileged information and data was, and wondered about how I repaid my obligation to my subjects. In the short run, the housestaff resolved the problem of helplessness and indebtedness by the roles they cast for me. When housestaff demanded that I help out by wheeling the chart rack, opening dressings, acting as a group memory, they provided me a means to cope with my own helplessness and assuage my guilt at the same time that they incorporated me into the group. While I was in the field, my involvement in the group resolved for me the problems I experienced as an indebted guest.

These problems reemerged when I left the field and began writing up the report. I saw much that was wrong in surgery, but what I saw emerged against the background of dedicated people working tirelessly at very difficult and complex tasks. What if what I reported was harmful to those that made the account possible? I had the problems of balancing my universal obligations to sociological analysis to my particular obligations to my research subjects. Unfortunately for me, I could not expect anyone to point the way by the everyday roles they cast me in. One thing I did was not begin writing immediately on leaving the field. Before drafting this report, I let the freshness of the experience recede somewhat so that I would not be overwhelmed by the memory of my relations with particular individuals. Second, when recording field notes, I made every attempt to keep my description of events as behavioral as possible, and my recording of conversations as verbatim as possible. At all times, I tried to keep "in situ" analysis separate from my field descriptions. I kept two different categories of field notes: (1) a log of happenings, conversations, and conferences; and (2) a separate running analysis. In this way I was later able to identify for and correct problems that resulted from overraport or over-indebtedness. By this procedure, I would see where the data confirmed, or failed to support, my analyses. There is in fieldwork always the problem of selective data collecting and analysis that might harm one's subjects. Any definitive resolution to this problem awaits more sophisticated, but at the same time unobtrusive, techniques of gathering field data. At the present, the length of time we spend in the field and our own intellectual integrity is our only protection from this problem. Third, I shared my report with the surgeons upon its completion. We discussed areas of disagreement between our interpretations. In particular, they objected to the rhetoric of sociology; they saw my framing the problem with a deviance and social-control vocabulary as unnecessarily pejorative, but they accepted (even if they did not agree with or fully understand) my rationale. They agreed that I had most of the phenomenological description right, if not always the interpretations. However, where there were interpretive disagreements, the surgeons attributed them to my being a sociologist, and accepted my analysis as valid from my frame of reference. They suggested ways that I could better protect the anonymity and confidentiality of individuals. For example, at their request, I changed the pseudonyms I originally chose and excised all dates from my field materials. I resolved part of my debt by allowing the surgeons to observe me as a sociologist at work.

Overgeneralization is also a recurrent problem for field-workers at two levels. First, there is the danger that one particular event will become etched in the field-worker's memory as emblematic of the way action is organized in an environment. That is to say, field-workers may overgeneralize incidents and see them as representative of categories of action. Second, field-workers may overgeneralize from their particular sites to all other types of similar settings. In the first case, I avoided overgeneralization by making sure I had

at least two independently generated examples of the same phenomenon before I began to make inferences. My operating rule here was, as far as I can
see, not fundamentally different than those that survey researchers use to
ensure reliability in their studies. Also, I was very careful to follow particular incidents through many levels of social organization. For example, I was
able to test my inferences about normative error in the promotion meeting, where I observed the criteria attending surgeons use to judge the fit-
ness of housestaff for surgical careers. Throughout my fieldwork, I was very
careful to test observations in one context against those of another. On the
other hand, there are observations I made that did not find their way into the
fieldwork because I felt my inferential base was too thin. On one occasion I
watched a series of unexpected deaths and complications, which occurred in
quick succession, temporarily destroy the morale of Able Service. These occurred during the end of a rotation, while a chief resident was on vacation. I
developed an explanation which related the occurrence of failure and group
panic. However, during the rest of my fieldwork, I did not have the opportunity to observe another rash of failures. As a result, such speculations did not
find their way into the manuscript. As an aid to the reader, I have tried to indicate throughout the text where inferences are based on slim observation.

There is a second type of overgeneralization—generalization from the
specific case, Pacific Hospital, to hospitals that are not included in Pacific's
class. Pacific is a member of the medical elite. There are perhaps twenty
hospitals in this country with the same reputation for excellence that Pacific
has. I am confident that the description of controls at Pacific is one that fits
virtually all members of this class. I am also confident that I have described
and analyzed a professional "ideal type," an environment where the major
preoccupations have to do with the aesthetics and elegance of surgery, un-
contaminated by such mundane matters as fees, social networks to generate
referrals, and market pressures. How the system of social control I described
is modified in more modal settings is a question that deserves further research, as is the question of how comparable it is to the systems of social
control in other professions. These are questions that I am beginning to work
on now. There is certainly no intrinsic reason that fieldwork cannot be as cu-
mulative as any other area of sociology. The benefit of using a site like Pacific
as a starting point is that physicians there are quite self-conscious about their
place in the medical world, and make explicit reference to why they deserve
an esteemed place in the profession. Moreover, being so self-conscious, they
are eager to inculcate into their young recruits the values in which they believe so strongly. Attending surgeons see their trainees as extensions of them-

selves in many ways; one of these is that they expect the conduct of those whom they train to reflect honor and glory back on Pacific.

Out of the Field

One peculiarity of field research is that one discovers what one learns in the field often only after one has left the field. So, strangely, the most creative and fruitful periods of field research are those where the researcher steps back from his immersion in an alien world, takes stock, and decides where to go next. By alternating periods of total immersion with periods of analysis, the field-worker can avoid phenomenological fatigue, that is, the sense of "I've seen it all before," and can continually refine and sharpen the questions asked of a particular research. For this study, I normally spent two or three months in the field, full-time, recording my observations in as straightforward a manner as possible, left the field for two weeks to a month to analyze my data, and then returned with a greater sense of what I now knew and what I still had to learn about the conduct of surgeons. For example, after retreating from the field the first time, I discovered in my notes that surgeons treated some mistakes as normal occurrences, while other events were treated as quite extraordinary and unacceptable performances. But at that time, I did not know why one set of events was categorized by actors in one way and another was so differently treated. It was clear very early in the study that the seriousness of an error was not determined by a set of precedent variables such as the patient's age or social status, nor was it determined by such antecedent variables as what happens to the patient. An error's seriousness was related only incidentally to the patient and his condition. On the other hand, seriousness was related in a very direct fashion to the attending's reaction. Discovering this, I felt reassured and at the same time I knew nothing, since I did not know what determined the attending's reaction.

My first immersion in the field in some sense determined the direction of most of my subsequent observation, as I tried to unravel what the bases of attending evaluation were, how clear these were to housestaff, and how widely they were shared among all members of the team. A dialectic of immersion and reflection that began the first day I arrived on the surgery wards at Pacific—and which I am sure is not completed—allowed me a continuous sense of discovery. It is worth noting, for instance, that I did not discover quasi-normative errors until after I left the field entirely. I had not seen while in the field so clearly how the lines of cleavage among the ranks were structured. In turn, my new understanding that there were two distinct types of normative error forced me to revise my conclusions about the social controls in surgical training by allowing me to see some of the ways its ethical content is undermined. I also gained a new respect for what it means "to let your field data speak to you." There are any number of things about the field that one discovers only by not being there. I discovered the "charisma" of surgery, not in the hospital but at parties and other social events. Being a sociologist does not normally make one the center of attention; however, being a sociologist who studies surgeons does. As my research progressed, I was struck by the almost primal awe my friends and acquaintances had for surgeons. Normally sophisticated urban dwellers with Simmel's (1970) blasé attitude would literally beg for details about what surgeons were really like, about what went on in operating rooms, about what their doctors were really like. It occurred to me that I had, through my close association with them, borrowed part of the surgeons' charisma. Seeing that the surgeons' charisma was not just some dramaturgic creation in organized social settings helped me understand how the surgeons' autonomy was as great and unchecked as it was. It also made me see that this was not simply a result of surgeons' behavior but was also nurtured by patients' needs and desires. Cocktail party curiosity also alerted me to how little people know about the medical care they receive, how few people have ever been in an operating room as an observer, and how powerful and coexistent are the contradictory impulses both to glorify and to degrade the surgeon. (Cocktail parties also taught me of the need for circumspection and tact, which I shall comment on below.)

Unfortunately, I did not learn as much from leaving the field as I might have, because I did not keep a careful record of why I chose to leave the field at the times I did. I assume that had I been as clear as I might about my comings and goings, about what was going on in the field that would make me willing or eager to leave, then I might have gained some greater understanding than I have about the surgeon's life space. I know there were days when I had to force myself to go to the hospital, and other days when I grabbed at any straw as an excuse for a breather. But when and why these feelings intensified at the times they did, I do not know. Such knowledge is of more than private psychodynamic interest (though it is of that also), for it helps make clear what strains field-workers are subject to in medical settings, how they can better prepare themselves, and how they can be better supervised. The end result from such understanding would be more valid and reliable monographs, less likely to be subject to any "observer effect."

Data, Confidentiality, and the Field-Worker

I indicated above that I learned some lessons at cocktail parties about circum-spection. In a literal sense, this is not true; but social situations presented me with a sticky problem. When I was in the middle of the field, disguising the place and principals of my study was not as easy as it is in this report. I was always aware when I spoke that others knew those I spoke of, and that a too-loose tongue could hurt me and them in many untold ways. Since I promised my subjects confidentiality and anonymity, the "cover story" I de-vised to manage social situations was as consequential as the one I devised to manage field introductions. Only by assuring confidentiality and anonymity could I satisfy my subjects that my study would be within the bounds of cur-rent medical ethics. Both promises present some dilemmas, however.

First, I could not ever be sure that some enterprising person would not be able to figure out my place and principals. Essentially, confidentiality and anonymity were the promises I made but I had little control over their fulfill-ment. There have been recent debates about whether field-workers should go to the bother of making general "covering names" for their sites, and whether they should disguise their subjects. It seems to me that such ficti-tious names do more than provide confidentiality and anonymity: they high-light the generalized features of our descriptions and minimize the particu-larized aspects. To my mind, this aspect of naming is even more important in some ways than confidentiality and anonymity in that it creates a fieldwork literature rather than a description of specific places; for example, Bellevue, Long Island Jewish Hospital, Johns Hopkins.

Others have advocated that to make fieldwork more rigorous and to dis-play our methodology more openly, we should open our notebooks to the curious. Such procedure would allow others to see how we manipulate our data and fit the canons of science in general. Such a proposal troubles me because, as a sociologist, I gathered litigable material from subjects who trusted me. As a sociologist, I have no legal right to claim a privileged or confidential relationship with my subjects; my notes are subpoenable. If I opened my notebooks in the manner necessary to make clear the operations I performed on my data, I risk having those notebooks put to uses other than those I approve of by people whose motives I may distrust for reasons I think are less than just. Involved here is a difficult problem: how to afford my subjects and myself enough protection so that we feel comfortable doing the study, at the same time displaying my data in a way that assures others of the validity and reliability of my research. I have indicated for the reader what I have done to satisfy myself of this report's accuracy. For the moment, I suggest that this—along with giving and receiving adequate supervision—is the best I can do.

Conclusion

As a research method, fieldwork yields results that often are phenomenologically rich, theoretically provocative, and practically useful. The major liability with this research method is that there are no procedures internal to the techniques of field research itself that control validity and reliability. The major data-gathering technique that the researcher utilizes is his relationship with his subjects. For better or worse the rules that govern relationships are less precise, harder to articulate, and more complexly interwoven with other normative systems than the rules that govern, for example, item construction on a questionnaire. By the same token, the field-worker's sampling procedures and the manipulations he performs on his data are often left unexplained. Clearly it is not that field-workers do not gather data by rules, sample from everyday life in a complex fashion, or manipulate their data. Rather, it is the case that to state what the rules are requires statements of such generality that they are of little use in any particular setting. The reason for this is not hard to understand: our subjects are never simply subjects. They also occupy a variety of other roles and the rules that govern relationships, for example, with physicians are different than those that govern relationships with heroin addicts. This inherent variation imposes on the field-worker his special obligation. The field-worker must describe the role relations that he had with his subjects as clearly and honestly as he can. The field-worker must describe how he avoided overinvolvement or on what occasions he succumbed to it, how he avoided overgeneralizing, and how he avoided over-indebtedness to his subjects. A clear statement of the social matrix out of which the field materials emerged allows the reader to judge validity and reliability for himself. At the same time, it has the added benefit of providing comparable accounts of the fieldwork experience which allows us to see what is general to a researcher's relations to his subject and what is particularly his own.

TEN

An Ethnographer's Apology,
a Bioethicist's Lament

THE SURGEON AND THE SOCIOLOGIST REVISITED

After rereading his novella *A River Runs Through It*, Norman MacLean said that he would not change so much as a comma. Having read that work, I agree. Beyond that, I envy MacLean his certainty. After periodically rereading my own work, there is much that I would change. I remember that just before *Forgive and Remember* was published I obsessed about the possibility that I got this or that detail wrong. I then went on to magnify my obsessions: What if none of the interpretation was correct? What if I used my data to construct a plausible delusional system? I knew that I had written a tight, coherent argument. But I also knew that nothing is so coherent as the ranting of a paranoid. I was not particularly reassured by the kind words from my informants who looked at the manuscript and commented on how much I had gotten right. In fact, such appreciative comments merely fueled my panic. I had not created an independent delusion of a specialized social world; I was not that creative. What I had done was more pedestrian; I had simply bought into and crudely represented the surgeons' collectively organized and professionally shared delusional system. Irrational as they were, such were my fears on the eve of publication.

Chapter 10 was originally published as Charles L. Bosk, "An Amended Appendix— An Ethnographer's Apology, A Bioethicist's Lament: The Surgeon and The Sociologist Revisited," in *Forgive and Remember: Managing Medical Failure*, 2nd edition. (Chicago: University of Chicago Press, 2003), 215–35.

I had always been taught that a good fieldwork account contained insights unpleasant to subjects, the dirty professional secrets that subjects would prefer to keep hidden, the ass end of the sacred. There was, I also had been taught, a similarity in fieldwork and psychoanalysis—both make the latent manifest—the truth of what is brought to light is indexed by the amount of resistance these new insights provoke. The implication of these beliefs for me, as an ethnographer, was that if my subjects approved of what I had written, if they identified with it, if they liked it, then I must not have penetrated too deeply into their world. And so it went. On the eve of publication, I still went back and forth between two conflicting fears. Either I made it all up or I just stated the obvious. In the end, I comforted myself with the thought that though veracity was a goal, though a commitment to getting the facts right was what separated ethnography from fiction, I still had told a good story, a useful story. I began to think that maybe what was important was not literal or even interpretative truth, which I now saw as an elusive goal. What was important was to create a version of reality that would in Levi-Strauss's memorable formula be "good to think with."

With this conviction, I suppose I could claim some sort of foresight. I was a post-modernist ahead of the curve. I would gladly claim credit if I could. But the conviction that a good story was the best that I could do felt much more like a face-saving rationalization than an epistemological belief. In any case, as an empirical sociologist, I saw a clear difference between believing that many interpretations of one reality were possible and believing that only multiple interpretations existed, none more authoritative than any other. The fact that in surgery people acted and as a consequence people lived or died, professional actions were judged, residents and nurses were most likely to be found wanting, predisposed me to the "someone here has the power and authority to make decisions that matter" model of social life. The voice of unchallenged organizational authority in *Forgive and Remember* is, as the epilogue makes clear, the attending surgeon. I never directly challenged the authority of the attending surgeons in everyday decision making—it would have been the end of my study. I gave voice in the text to the residents' complaints, but constantly reminded the reader how unrewarding frontal assaults on authority are for floor nurses and residents. The grumblings that I give voice to were all expressed in settings and at times when attending surgeons were not present.

Even so, it is more than twenty years later, and I still find myself bothered not by the story I told but by two stories I chose not to tell. At the time, each of the two omissions that I am now about to remedy struck me as not just morally justifiable but as morally necessary. But with all the hindsight that a long stretch of time provides, I see that each omission had theoretical consequences for the story I told. Each blunted the interpretation, analysis, and critique of surgical training and professional socialization, shop-floor ethics, and professional social control embedded in the ethnographic account.

The first omission occurs in chapter five, "Climbing the Pyramid: Professional Control and Moral Identity." The chapter is an attempt to show how attending surgeons' everyday judgments of residents' performance exert a career influence. The chapter is described as a natural experiment testing the book's major hypothesis: namely that technical and judgmental errors were blameless while normative and quasi-normative errors were blameworthy. The chapter unfolds to show how this is the logic attendings use either to promote residents to the next level of training or to deny such promotion. The chapter "demonstrate[s] that the promotion decision is a presumptive moral licensing that provisionally admits or blackballs a subordinate from the fraternity of academic surgeons" (149).

In the chapter, only the behavior of residents is problematic. I do not stop to question whether the criteria, standards, rationalizations, or processes that attending surgeons employ might themselves be problematic. I also do not display any of the data that I collected that would allow others to raise these questions. The absence of such data is important. Ethnography is less good to think with if it does not provide a rich enough database to allow readers to frame alternatives, to disagree with authorial certainty, to see things differently. Here I am documenting how omissions made *Forgive and Remember* less good to think with. I edited my data, changed a critical fact (and I recognize that changing the facts contravenes some rather stringent ethical norms of science) and, in so doing, made my own work less rich. I did so in order to obey the canons, as I understood them, of ethnographic ethics.[1] What is offered here is offered in the spirit of correction and apology. This then is an act of self-revision; as such, it is not clear how much of this should be done in public. There is a thin line between improvement and indulgence. I tread it in the hope that, on balance, the discussion presented here falls on the positive side of the ledger.

Changing the Facts

I suppose the time has come to present what was initially misrepresented, to correct what was changed. In order to make the correction I need to present a large section of text. The following material describes the promotion meeting at which surgical faculty meet to decide the fate of second-year surgical residents:

> The faculty agreed as quickly as they did in Smith's case that a second candidate, Jones, lacked the technical skills necessary for a surgical career. But in this second case, they had grave doubts about whether Jones had any place in the medical profession at all. Jones combined technical maladroitness with an inability to admit mistakes and difficulties in communicating with patients and staff. This had led on occasion to small correctable errors growing into catastrophes.

> Dr. Gray opened discussion of Jones by reporting: "Jones has had a lot of problems over the last fifteen months. This morning I talked with him and told him that an inability to communicate with peers and patients was not a quality we were looking for in our residents. I suggested to him that he meet with Dr. Cantor in psychiatry to discuss whatever personal problems he has before he makes any plans to continue his career in any capacity. He was quite adamant that he needed no help and that he wanted to be a surgeon." Dr. Grant said: "I did not know what to make of Dr. Jones his first few days on our service, but I have reluctantly come to the conclusion that this man is sick. I don't trust him around my patients." An attending asked, "How do you mean sick— physically or mentally?" Dr. Arthur answered, "Mentally. He's off his rocker. Totally out to lunch. He needs help and he needs it quick. The question is not whether we should keep him, but whether he should finish out the year. In my mind, I wonder if he's on drugs." Dr. Gray then said: "As I said before when I gave him the option of seeing Dr. Cantor, he was totally opposed to it." Dr. Grant added: "There is no doubt he needs help. Yesterday in clinic he was really around the bend. He couldn't focus on patients. You could not have a conversation with him. He couldn't deal with anything." Dr. Peters commented that "it doesn't sound like much has changed over the course of a year. Maybe he has a brain tumor." Dr. Ross said: "If he has a problem, I don't think we could in good conscience let him go without offering him help. I think we have a responsibility to see that he gets proper care. But our responsibility to our patients comes first. If there is any doubt about his stability, we cannot continue to let him see patients." Dr. Gray then summarized the comments about Jones by saying: "Then we are all agreed. Not only will Jones not be offered a position, but he will not be allowed to return to duty

until he is investigated by someone in neuropsychiatry" ([Surgery Department Faculty] Meeting).

The attendings felt some responsibility for Jones as a person under their care. However, Jones' breaches were so consistent and so consistently denied by Jones that immediate expulsion was necessary. Unlike Smith, Jones was not a tracking problem. He was a total problem that attendings wished to rid themselves of entirely by shifting responsibility to the psychiatry department.

The contrast between the handling of Smith and Jones supports my argument about the differences between technical and normative error and also suggests inherent limits to professional control (156–57).

What the analysis nowhere suggests is that those inherent limits have to do with biases in applying available standards to mete out appropriate sanctions. In the above, I refer to Jones as a gendered person ("him, he, his, this man") a total of thirty-four times in the space of one manuscript page. All of these references are deliberately misleading; Jones was the sole female in the cohort of surgical residents I observed.

When drafting the manuscript, I did not think twice about changing Jones's gender. I had promised my subjects confidentiality and anonymity. There was no way that I could think of to keep Jones a woman and honor that pledge.[2] So "she" became "he," and the analysis proceeded without missing a beat—a study of standards and their use. I raised no questions about whether those standards that reinforce group norms and that are so transparently fair on their face are ever used in ways that reinforce existing prejudices and inequities. The fact that I shared the attendings' discomfort with Jones, as did virtually all of her peers, helped blind me to the impact of gender. Jones was difficult to talk to; among the residents she was the one who avoided me the most and who volunteered the least. And what she did volunteer, I often had difficulty understanding. Beyond that, if Jones did distrust me—and I always sensed that she did—for me that was further proof of her limitations. After all, I was different than the male attendings and residents. I knew that, and I was not yet wise enough to see why Jones might quite reasonably not know it as well. I never gathered data that dealt squarely with how Jones understood the effect of her gender on her career as a surgical resident. Jones was silent with me and I did not know how to break through that silence. As a result, I never gave voice to her complaints, never allowed her voice to challenge directly the authoritative voice of attending authority.

I'd like to be able to say that today, anonymity and confidentiality be damned, I'd never change gender again. I recognize now that it is too important a determinant of behavior to ignore. Unfortunately, this is a goal that is hard to uphold. Before the publication of *All God's Mistakes,* one of the genetic counselors complained that her identity was too thinly veiled (I had kept gender and ethnicity correct when assigning a pseudonym). She wanted her name changed to "Bill Smith." I fussed and fumed but I did what she asked. I did not think I had any choice. I had promised her confidentiality and anonymity and I felt I had to do anything she felt necessary to assure them, even if I thought the request unreasonable. But the two instances differ—in one case, a subject asked for protection; in the other, I provided it without being asked. In a peculiar way, the change involving Jones offered more protection to the surgeons of Pacific Hospital than it did to Jones. I don't know if Jones felt protected or if she desired anonymity. In fact, for the longest time, I didn't know what became of Jones. After the faculty meeting at which it was decided that she have coercive psychotherapy before resuming her duties, I never saw her again. Neither did anyone else. Faculty and residents alike knew only that she had moved out of her apartment. No one knew where she was. She had disappeared without a trace, as powerful an indicator of her social isolation within the group as one could imagine. When I first had the idea of a second edition, I decided to interview Jones and Carter to see how they viewed the events that *Forgive and Remember* chronicles. I knew where to find Carter and I set about to track down Jones. What I found on the internet was a recent obituary that indicated that Jones had risen to great prominence in the world of emergency medicine. This confirmed that there was something amiss both in the original assessment of her performance and my unquestioning acceptance of it.

So now, over twenty years later, I look at the text and wonder how I could have left gender out. A good many of the points feminists make about male domination are present in the brief vignette: Dr. Jones is placed in the sick role and seen as a candidate for psychiatric care (She's "totally out to lunch," "around the bend"). One physician even suggests, somewhat illogically since there had been no progression of symptoms, that "maybe she has a tumor." Another suggests that Dr. Jones is "on drugs." At this point in the 1970s, she would not have been alone among the surgical residents at Pacific if she engaged in sporadic, episodic recreational drug use. Who knows—perhaps that activity would have had the beneficial effect of connecting her with her peers in a mutually shared activity.

I have no doubt that changing genders theoretically impoverished my discussion of the moral order of surgical training. I also have no doubt that under the circumstances I had little choice but to switch Jones's gender. As a result, no matter how alive to the nuances of gender I might have been, no matter how alive I was to why Jones had so much trouble communicating (and I was not as aware as I think I should have been), I was not free to share this knowledge with readers. In the text of *Forgive and Remember,* I go on at great length describing how much informal communication and bonding goes on in the surgeons' locker room and the attached lounge. I detail in the text how the atmosphere of the locker room assuages and blurs for a time the hierarchy of an academic surgical service. In the locker room, surgeons relax, war stories are shared, and group solidarity is reinforced. Such moments were not planned; they did not happen according to a schedule or every time surgeons changed from street clothes into surgical greens. In fact, what is magical and wondrous about such moments, what intensifies the shared intimacy, is their randomness. They are not in any ordinary way planned for or predicted but they do happen. Predictable or not, such moments were not shared by Jones. She dressed with the nurses. She never hung around in the male lounge. Jones may have been unable to communicate because she did not get many opportunities. Beyond that, I realize now that without doubt Jones worked in a "hostile environment" and that such environments are, arguably, an indicator of harassment.

In multiple ways, I was more a member of the team than Jones: I shared a locker room with the guys, played squash with them, slept in the same on-call room (Jones had a separate room), drank beer with them, shared lewd comments about the nurses, and swapped smutty stories. I was one of the boys and Jones was not. Here it is perhaps important to note that Jones and I were often misidentified by those who did not know our actual social identities. A sociologist in white lab coat and surgical greens, I was often thought to be a surgical resident. A surgical resident in lab coat and scrubs, Jones was often thought to be a nurse.

On those occasions when I have discussed with others my discomfort now about switching Jones' identity then, I have been told that I am being unnecessarily hard on myself. I am judging my behavior by standards that did not apply at the time. While I think this is largely true, it is cold comfort and it points to a larger problem. Whenever I ask myself, How is ethnography justified as other than a privileged and self-indulgent professional activity? and What should ethnography do? part of my answer is always that ethnography provides data with which to critique the fit between our actions and our ideals. If we are trapped in the values of the everyday, how do we do this effectively? Beyond that, when we alter our data to protect our subjects, how do we know that the data we alter is not critical? What is an innocent change and what is not? (Davis 1991; Chambers 1999). My problem with changing Jones's gender is that it makes the critique I did not make impossible for others to make. To say that I was a prisoner of my times seems too convenient, too exculpatory. After all, it was not as if there were no critiques in the late 1970s of the patriarchal excesses of medicine. It seems to me that what happened was more complex—a conflict with one sort of value (anonymity and confidentiality) led me to betray, wittingly and unwittingly, another kind of value (commitment to an egalitarian society).

The Second Omission

Above I suggested that I was sure that Jones was a victim of gender harassment because she worked in a "hostile environment". This is a serious charge and I do not make it lightly. Yet there is very little in the text that would support such a charge. I do indicate that the work of being a surgical resident is stressful. But I generally paint a picture that has that stress flowing quite naturally out of the intrinsic problems of doing surgery at a major academic medical center—difficult cases that lesser surgeons will not touch, the shortage of ancillary services that routinely plagues academic medical centers, and the violent trauma and tragedy that are all too common in the inner city.

There was a dimension to the stress that I quite consciously chose not to mention. That dimension was the hectoring, often abusive behavior of senior surgeons. One of the reasons that I am so sure that Jones was harassed is that verbal harassment was a rather routine event for all residents, regardless of their gender. Senior surgeons, many of whom had their first experience as battlefield surgeons, believed that residency was a stress test. Part of surgical training for them was recreating the battlefield conditions they felt were so critical in developing their own excellence. So when the world did not throw enough problems in the fledgling surgeon's way, then the senior surgeons occasionally felt free to create some on their own.[3] The most spectacular incident of a "private stress test" that I observed did not find its way into the text of *Forgive and Remember*. Before I explain, let me describe.

I have been sifting through old field notes for more than a few hours over a couple of days now. While this unexpected stroll has had rewards all its own, the time-stained foolscap that I had been seeking has eluded me. This baffled me. There were more field notes in manila folders than I remember writing, each recording encounters that I had long ago forgotten. Yet missing were notes I recall writing that described an incident I remember as if it had happened yesterday. But the notes describing the particular incident that I wish to present are nowhere to be found among all the other notes that so meticulously describe people, places, and incidents that I no longer remember witnessing.[4] I am about to describe, in single-spaced indented form to signal typographically that it is from field notes, an incident which occurred over a quarter of century ago but which is being written up in the present. In texture and detail, the note is a pallid copy of the lost original. I suppose this takes me from the realm of revision to the realm of creation. Empirically what I report here is an ethnographic urban legend that can't be verified. Anyway, here is something that happened that I cannot find in my notes; something, in other words, that I have no business reporting as data:

> I am late and not for the first time. I change alone in the locker room. As I change, I muse. I just have a white lab coat with adhesive tape covering its rightful owner's name. I do not have a hospital I.D. card. I have been at this fieldwork over a year. How come I have never been stopped as I move to and from restricted areas of the hospital alone—SICU, patient rooms, X-ray, supply closets, nurses' stations, doctors' lounges, E.R. treatment rooms, the O.R.? Once as I bolted from a toilet stall where I was taking notes and raced from the latrine without flushing or washing my hands, I was dressed down by an attending and given a lecture on proper hygiene. But, of course the very fact that he felt free to lecture me indicated that he never doubted that I belonged to one of Pacific Hospital's training programs. I suppose that early in the fieldwork I thought it necessary to take notes in a toilet stall indicated that I was not so confident that I legitimately belonged at Pacific as the attending who chastised me was. What kind of security system is it that can be breached by race and gender alone?[5] I wondered, how did the attendings, so intolerant of the residents' lateness, view mine?
>
> I raced into the operating room feeling, as always, slightly ridiculous in a green scrub suit, the bottoms of which I can never tie properly, paper booties, hairnet over a massive frizz, hastily tied mask, and fogged glasses. I enter operating room three looking for the Baker Team. They are in room two, I'm told. I enter room two from the scrub area. Dr Arthur greeted me with effusive sarcasm. Sarcasm itself was not unexpected, his taking special notice of my presence was. "Oh, good, the sociologist has joined us. How nice of you

to come, Bosk." He was hanging on the side, unscrubbed—The Homeless Surgeon—this too was unusual. Christian was performing the surgery. Carter was acting as his first assistant.

After a short pause, Dr. Arthur spoke to me again, "Have you done your Mother's Day shopping yet? Perhaps Dr. Christian [who is German] could make you a lampshade from the cuttings and trimmings today? You know, Christian, I haven't seen this much blood since your relatives greeted the chief rabbi of Berlin during the war."[6] Arthur went on like this for a while. After he failed to get a reaction from Christian or Carter or me (we are both Jewish), he moved on to others. He turned to the anesthesiologist (who is an Asian woman) and, invoking his experience as a field surgeon during the Korean War, made some derogatory comments about "slopes, gooks, and dinks." When Arthur failed to get more than a roll of the eyes from the anesthesiologist, he turned to his regular scrub nurse (who is black) and asked her, "Do you know how many times I had to practice this operation on blacks before they let me do it on whites?" The scrub nurse did not respond. Instead, she asked Christian if he was ready for some instrument or suture material. Failing to get a reaction, Arthur began to grumble about the pace of the surgery, then fell silent, and left the room as his residents prepared to close.

After the surgery was completed, after evening rounds were completed, I gathered with the residents in the cafeteria for dinner. Josh Carter was fuming: "I couldn't believe Arthur today. Did you ever see a bigger jackass? I felt like slugging him." Christian said: "It's part of his making everything a stress test. You have to let it go in one ear and out the other." Carter then turned to me: "I'm not like Christian. I can't stand that shit. But it's part of what we have to put up with if we want to get through this program. We have to shut up and take stuff like that. Look, I'm Jewish and so are you, I don't know how you felt but I felt like walking out of the operating room. I don't really want to scrub with him anymore. I don't know if I can take it. But what choice do I have? If I say anything, I'm gone. So you have to shut up and take it. But did you ever see a bigger shithead than Arthur today?"

Truth was I probably had not. Arthur was a complex character, insulting one day, charming the next. With Arthur, one never quite knew what to expect. One did know that unless one met his standards, one's rotation on his service was likely to be a very close approximation of a living hell. Further, even if one met his standards but was on his wrong side—as Carter was to become—then the standards changed in such a way that one could not meet them. It was on the Baker Service, after repeatedly watching Arthur in action, that I developed the concept of quasi-normative error.

> Quasi-normative errors are eccentric and attending-specific. Each attending has certain protocols that he[sic] and he[sic] alone follows. A subordinate who does not follow these rules mocks his superordinate's authority; his behavior is a claim that his judgment is as adequate as his superior's; and even though in no absolute sense can one claim that a mistake has been made, a subordinate who makes a quasi-normative error risks his reputation as a trustworthy recruit (61).

Later in the text, in the chapter already discussed with regard to Jones, "Climbing the Pyramid," I spent a considerable amount of time analyzing the case of Josh Carter. In the promotion meeting in which Jones was determined to be unfit to continue, Carter was said to be an example of the head-strong type of resident who made quasi-normative errors and, as a result, failed to be retained in the training program. In the chapter, Carter's problems were seen entirely as a consequence of Carter's own doings. During the meeting, attendings praised Carter as an individual of great promise, talent, and ability. At the same time, he was criticized for being on occasion unreliable, untrustworthy, slovenly, and churlish. When I mentioned to an attending after the meeting that some of the criticism of Carter seemed to me petty, he responded, "Just because it's trivial doesn't mean it is unimportant."

Although I was certainly aware of them, for I had witnessed them, I did not discuss anywhere in the text of *Forgive and Remember* the provocations under which Carter and his peers worked. By not doing so I undermined my own intent in developing the concept of quasi-normative error. My intent, as I understood it at the time, was to show that the world of surgery was a highly authoritarian one and that that authority had a defect—it was occasionally eccentric, arbitrary, and capricious. Yet by not showing the degree to which Carter and others were baited, I lodge the defect not in authority itself, but in underlings who are too dim to discern its workings.

Looking back, I think I can see why I might have done so. I wanted my work to read differently than other sociological accounts of the time which seemed to engage routinely and somewhat unreflexively in doctor bashing. I felt that to present the most extreme examples of boorish behavior from my field notes would draw attention away from the book's central thesis—that in surgical education technical norms are subordinated to moral ones. I worried that parading Arthur's excesses—and Arthur, when I knew him, was a man of excesses—would draw attention away from the serious side of surgery and, for that matter, of Arthur. In the end, Arthur's colleagues tolerated his excesses because they recognized that they stemmed from his commitment to excellence and they recognized as well how closely his own performance as a surgeon approached that excellence. At the same time, Arthur's excellence was very much a tightly wound coil; picking at any loose end was a risky and explosive activity. In the end, I behaved like Arthur's colleagues—I forgave him his trespasses. I was appalled and I was charmed. I was only skilled enough as an ethnographic draftsman to present the charmed side.

But there are two problems with this that I now clearly see. First, my behavior, as well as the behavior of Arthur's colleagues, challenges my central thesis about the dominance of normative over technical standards. After all, Arthur's behavior was a normative abomination. We would not tolerate it now. I should not have been silent about it then. To be fair to myself, the text makes the point quite plainly that senior surgeons are not subject to the same rules as residents. It does talk about variation in attending style. But I think that this is all too coy, too clever by half. Second, I feel uneasy about Jones and Carter. The text makes them out to be social incompetents of a sort. They are too simple to figure out the rules of the game. Their problems then are of their own making. Yet this is neither entirely so nor entirely fair. So, I sometimes feel guilty about my treatment of these two residents. There are two dimensions of this guilt worth mentioning here. Most obviously, there is the breaking of generational ranks. I betrayed my peers. In addition, I sided with the aggressor. I know that this is a common enough thing to do in a total institution. All the same I'm not proud.

Some Concluding Remarks, or Why I Told These Stories

Why tell these stories now, so long after they occurred? Why sully Arthur's reputation as a surgeon or my own as a field-worker? Absolution might be one reason that I am choosing now "to put on a hairshirt," but I do not think it is the principal one despite the quite obvious cathartic effect for me of what I have written. I tell these stories now to point out some difficulties embedded in storytelling for didactic purposes. I certainly wanted to emphasize that what stories we choose to tell from our field notes and how we choose to tell them have important consequences. But there is more: I want the re-visioning of the occupational ethics of surgeons presented here to trace some of the fuzzy boundary between the established domain of cultural ethnography and the emerging one of narrative bioethics. I want to suggest why ethnography is not as likely, as some have hoped, to save the life of bioethics (Hoffmaster 1992).

In writing *Forgive and Remember*, one of my goals was social portraiture. The introduction to *Forgive and Remember* sets two goals for "analytical" ethnography to follow. "First, I want to recapture and refine the old Durkheimian insight that each occupational group possesses its own morality. I want to specify what for the surgeon is the complex of ideas and sentiments, [the] ways of seeing and [of] feeling, [the] certain intellectual and moral framework distinctive of the entire group. . . . [Second I want to] inform policy by grounding it in a firm understanding of how participants construct their social worlds. It is only from this concrete understanding of the present practical order that any changes in the existing interactional politics of social control can be negotiated" (5–6). *Forgive and Remember* is medical sociology, an ethnographic description of a professional group's "occupational morals." It is not neutral about those morals; suggestions for improving them are found in the conclusion. On the one hand, in researching and writing *Forgive and Remember*, I strained to provide as detached, neutral, and objective an account as possible. Yet, on the other hand, I quite clearly fell short of this goal: with all the talk of "the moral order," "normative codes," and "blameworthy and blameless error," *Forgive and Remember* has a point of view; it can just as easily be read as applied social ethics as empirical social science, as prescriptive and normative as descriptive and empirical.

With these alternative readings in my mind, I presented the two omissions as a device for showing how problematic using ethnographic data for narrative ethics is, for discussing how different the role of bioethicist is from that of ethnographer, and for suggesting some guidelines for writing ethnographies that are "good to think with" either as a social scientist or bioethicist. Before moving on to those tasks, I need to clarify how I assess each of the omissions. The switching of gender, transforming Jones from her to him, strikes me now as a blameworthy error. The error is blameworthy for any number of reasons but most notably, because it makes the text less "good to think with." The very absence of women from the ranks of either attending surgeons or residents should have served as a clue that something worth discussing was out of kilter in the social world whose ethics I was describing. At the same time, I see leaving out the second omission—Arthur's ethnic, religious, and racial slurs—as trivial. I had provided more than enough evidence to suggest that Arthur was difficult to work for, easy to anger, and arbitrary in his judgments. I had also provided more than enough evidence that these faults were not Arthur's alone among senior surgeons, as well as evidence that residents found that the conditions of their employ were stressful. Leaving out the incident in the operating room did not make the ethnography any less good to think with. Including it, however, might have had that effect. It was so startling, so beyond the ordinary, and so offensive that the real danger existed that this behavioral outlier would skew the interpretation of the data. The incident was probably the single most offersive scene I observed during my year and a half of observation. My own sense of propriety, decorum, and fairness suggested to me that I would not want some observing other to hold up for inspection my most offensive professional behavior over the same time period.[7]

If that is so, why tell the second tale now? First, as a simple discursive strategy, the second vignette reinforces the point of the first: if the conditions that the men worked under included such coarse verbal harassment, then imagine what things must have been like for the women. For this point, I did not have direct evidence. Jones, remember, was a socially isolated woman in a group of men. She trusted me and spoke with me no more than she did with any of the other males around. At that time, I had not honed my own skills well enough to talk with a subject as marginalized and as vulnerable as Jones. Nor had I mastered ethnographic technique well enough to skillfully display reports of what did not happen, what was never observed, what was not asked and answered. So the second omission is told here to make the point of the first omission creditable: that had I paid attention to gender I might have noticed that the operation and application of quasi-normative standards undermines the formal fairness of the normative order of surgical training.

There is a second reason to remedy both omissions now. We have known for quite some time that ethnographic narratives are socially constructed, that they are told this way rather than that, that they privilege some voices rather than others. I have also said that the unchallenged voice of authority in the original version of *Forgive and Remember* is the attending surgeon. The previous chapter discussed some of the changes that have occurred now that the voice of attending authority is no longer quite so unchallenged. In this commentary, I want to suggest some natural troubles of ethics presented as ethnography or ethnography presented as ethics.

Framing this as a discussion at the boundary between narrative ethics and cultural ethnography imperfectly reframes it as a discussion between cultural insiders and outsiders. By and large those that practice any brand of narrative ethics base their claims to expertise, their special purchase on affairs, to some sort of "insider" status. By the same token, those who produce ethnographies of medicine base their claims to expertise, their special purchase on affairs, on their "outsider" status: lacking any stake in immediate outcomes permits continued neutrality, makes objective observation and analysis possible.

When I began the research for *Forgive and Remember,* I was an outsider at Pacific Hospital. Not only that, I was fairly certain that by the time the research was published, I would no longer be at Pacific. I would only have a few sentimental ties to Pacific Hospital's Department of Surgery. At the beginning of the research, I was an outsider who knew nothing of hospitals or of residency training. As the research went on, I learned things; and, as I learned things, I became more of an "insider," but there was always a "responsibility barrier"—I never had to make decisions and do things on behalf of others. As the research progressed, I developed relationships, made friends, and built up obligations. These all affected what stories I chose to tell and how I chose to tell them. In my own eyes, I was there to reveal how some of the backstage of surgery was connected to its public presentation. That became the general narrative guideline (save for Jones's gender) for constructing *Forgive and Remember.* On rereading the text, I am struck at what I chose to leave out the first time around, and the cool detached tone through which events are narrated, judgments made, and solutions proposed.

Narrative ethics is generally practiced by insiders in health care. Some are employed in hospitals in other clinical roles, some are hired purely for their expertise as ethicists to sit on hospital committees, provide in-service continuing and public education, contribute to research, and consult on difficult cases. In this work they develop relationships, make friends, juggle multiple responsibilities, and build up obligations. All of this work is done in an organizational environment in which strong professional norms of confidentiality exist and are routinely breached. If narrative ethicists wish to produce public ethnographic accounts of their work, they will need to trade on those relationships, betray some of those friendships, ignore some of their ethical obligations, and tread, however lightly, on those norms of confidentiality. The very work of telling stories, which may very well involve the public airing of some dirty organizational linen, may then transform insiders into outsiders in health care settings. Those with tales to tell may find themselves as frozen out of the everyday discourse as Jones was. This, then, may compromise their effectiveness as clinical workers in other domains, ethics committee members, or consultants.

All of this is to say that the intersection of ethnography, narrative, and ethics is vexed. The space between objective description and involved activity is closer than we might think if we are looking in the rearview mirror alone.

Ethnographers cannot retreat from studies of contested ethical situations. Our credentials as outsiders or insiders need to be continually negotiated and renegotiated. We need to think more complexly than we have about where the line that separates observer effect and the legitimate exercise of expertise is, how we will know we have crossed it, and how we will know when such crossings are not just permissible but compulsory. Narrative ethicists also have to think about the tradeoffs in their work as well, about when to argue and when to let go, and when to make a public issue of a private trouble.[8] For both ethnographers and narrative ethicists, how much of the backstage to reveal is a recurring question. How each answers that question is a function of how each defines the professional, the public, and the collective dimension of their role responsibilities. For cultural ethnographers as for narrative ethicists, social obligations and a sense of skill at meeting them spring from self-definition and from the paired questions: Why am I here and what am I doing?

The body of this chapter is a telling of stories I chose not to tell once upon a time. I pulled my punches even though I had no institutional interests to safeguard, no individuals I needed to protect, and no agenda that I sought to promote. Even with that, as a moral tale, an example of applied ethics, *Forgive and Remember* is a thickly described, thin story. The thick description is in the everyday account of the resident's life and professional vulnerabilities. The thin story is the account that does not more strongly question all the prerogatives claimed in the name of attending authority. This defect also suggests a remedy for those that engage in some form of applied ethics, whether ethnographic or narrative, theoretic or applied. We need to ask ourselves how many voices we have allowed to speak and how many hidden presumptions we have questioned. One mode of doing this for both ethnographers and narrative ethicists is to revisit our work from time to time and ask, How would we have acted differently, what story would we tell this time?

Works Cited

Bosk, Charles L. 1992. *All God's Mistakes: Genetic Counseling in a Pediatric Hospital.* Chicago: University of Chicago Press.

———. 2001. "Irony, Ethnography, and Informed Consent." In *Bioethics in Social Context,* edited by Barry C. Hoffmaster. Philadelphia: Temple University Press, 199–220.

Chambers, Tod. 1999. *The Fiction of Bioethics: Cases as Literary Texts.* New York: Routledge.

Davis, Dena. 1991. "Rich Cases: The Ethics of Thick Description." *Hastings Center Report* 21:12–17.

Notes

1. To speak of this under a rubric as ancient and formulaic as canons of ethics is a misrepresentation in the extreme of how I thought about the omissions at the time. I did not think about these omissions in a way as systematic and organized as invoking canons of ethics suggests. At the time, each omission seemed reasonable and necessary—as time has passed, and as we shall read in but a moment, I now think one of the omissions was justifiable and the other not.

2. Years later, when I first discussed this gender switch with colleagues, one asked, "Why not keep Jones a woman and make another resident one as well?" I thought it a good question with a ready answer. The question itself was a sign of how times had changed. The fact that that alternative never occurred to me says something about the gender composition of surgical training programs at the time of my fieldwork. I did not think about this option because the notion of two women in such a small program strained credulity.

3. To be fair, there was a great deal of variation here. Some senior surgeons never harassed, embarrassed, abused, bullied, or treated their residents with disrespect. Other senior surgeons rarely missed the opportunity. If that formulation is too strong, then perhaps it is more accurate to say that very little inhibited their attack impulses. It is worth noting that the more mild-mannered surgeon often had nothing but contempt for his, and now sometimes her, more histrionic peers. Whatever feelings the theatrical attending created among his colleagues, they suffered in silence. I never heard one senior surgeon correct or confront another. But, then, this is probably not the kind of activity in which two senior surgeons would engage in front of the novice outsider.

   Additionally, I suppose, one might argue that *Forgive and Remember* was written a long time ago and that surgeons no longer behave in any of these ways. The abusive behavior I am about to describe no longer takes place. That I think is true. But, then again, I chose not to include the incident that I am about to describe because it was so unrepresentative. However I recently have had occasion to interview all faculty and residents in six neurosurgical training programs. Reports of the total demise of the dramatically hectoring surgeon are exaggerated.

4. The very fact that the notes describe so much that I have forgotten seems strange to me. When I was doing the fieldwork, recording the notes certainly felt like a needless chore, a species of academic ritualism—"how could I ever forget this?" I thought. Going back over the forgotten notes somehow vindicated the importuning of my teachers at the time and justifies my current nagging of students in the field. The notes themselves index a

peculiar feature of fieldwork—we collect so much data and present so little of it.

5. To be truthful, I know that the lost note that I am reconstructing here did not have these musings about hospital security, which has considerably tightened in the wake of baby snatchings and assaults on hospital personnel and patients. Other notes, however, that I did not get to work into *Forgive and Remember,* do contain these musings and the toilet stall incident did actually occur on another day early in the fieldwork.

As an index of how things have changed since I did the fieldwork on surgeons, consider the following: I never received any formal administrative clearance to do the research for *Forgive and Remember,* had no consent form, and never really thought much of the ethics of proceeding without formal consent. When after reading the publication contract for *Forgive and Remember,* which held me liable for any legal actions consequent to publication, I suggested to my editor that the hospital attorney review the manuscript, the attorney was surprised that the research had been done but not unhappy with the result.

Of course, clearance and consent, as I later found out, are not much of a protection—for the researcher at least. (In truth, they are not intended to protect the researcher.) I had both for *All God's Mistakes* (Bosk 1992). Nonetheless my physician-subjects tried to block publication and threatened a lawsuit. In this second case, the hospital attorney was less surprised and less delighted by the appearance of a manuscript.

6. In the previous note, I indicated that the "reconstructed" note above contained materials that I was certain were not in the original. Here I should add that I am certain that these words were spoken in just this way. Much as I have tried to forget, to repress, these words, I have never had much success. But without the original note, you'll just have to take my word for it.

7. Beyond all that, the thought occurs that I did not find extreme verbal abuse by authority shocking or extraordinary. It was certainly part of the all-male public high school that I attended. Coaches on any team that I played on indulged in it quite frequently. Faculty at the college that I attended were not shy about dressing students down in class. I think that I expected senior surgeons to be verbally abusive. I was no more shocked by this than I would have been by an abusive army drill instructor. This kind of verbal abuse was not an unusual occurrence in male settings.

The very fact that I did not make much of verbal harassment is yet another reason why I did not make much of Jones's hostile work environment. After all, the hostility was not created by gender, it existed for everyone. However, as the lone woman, Jones may have experienced that verbal harassment differently than her male peers who were able to use each other for comfort and support.

8. This is Mills's formula and it remains a good one to think with. As everyday actors, those who practice clinical ethics need a keen sense of the sociological imagination. One way to assure such an imagination is collaborative projects that are multisited.

ELEVEN

A Monument of Silence

ON NOT GIVING UP DR. ARTHUR'S GHOST

After a long and overly detailed introduction—a thick description of the aftermath of one published attempt to provide a thick description of one social world—this chapter discusses one failed attempt to provide confidentiality and anonymity for subjects of a fieldwork study. I will discuss confidentiality and anonymity as a promise made to subjects, what the field-worker can do to fulfill that promise, what aspects of that promise over which the field-worker has no control, and what problems—some reasonably foreseeable and some more remote—are created when confidentiality and anonymity are breached. This discussion is motivated by my recently having received a solicitation from Pacific Hospital to contribute to the Dr. Arthur Memorial Lectureship in Surgical Education. The solicitation revealed some aspects of *Forgive and Remember* that I would rather had not been revealed, namely, which hospital was Pacific and which attending surgeon was Dr. Arthur.[1] My first reaction, after the momentary flattery of the free publicity and praise for my work that the solicitation contained passed, was, "I can't control everything. If the institution chooses to breach our agreement, it's not my problem." My second reaction was a form of outrage: "How dare they? Aren't our obligations reciprocal? Shouldn't they have asked before they did this? Don't I have any rights as to how my intellectual property is used?" Moving right along the chain of my affect, I then felt a dim sort of inarticulate worry. I knew something that the fundraisers at Pacific did not. To wit, as Van Maanen (1988) has remarked, the analysis of an experience in the field is never over, it is just finished for the time being, fixed in print now for this publication but not fixed forever—all interpretations, even those we publish, are provisional, open to endless revision.

And wouldn't you know it, as these things happen, at precisely the time the document that used my words to lionize Dr. Arthur arrived, I was finishing a manuscript much less flattering to him. That manuscript, which is the previous chapter in this volume, revisited the terrain of *Forgive and Remember*. In it, I described both how a gender switch that I made in the text to safeguard confidentiality and anonymity and how sensational incidents I suppressed in the original account blunted and obscured the theoretical argument of the eventual text. In particular, I was not able to discuss how stressful senior surgeons made the surgical workplace, on occasion, for residents and nurses. Dr. Arthur was, while not the only offender, the most florid and frequent one. This new paper highlighted the most spectacular breaches that he committed in my presence. As a result of my self-editing way back then, certain points I was trying to make about the arbitrary and capricious nature of authority got lost in the sweet reasonableness of arguments that I was making more forcefully. I had the strong impression that the fundraisers at Pacific, Arthur's former colleagues, and all of those who had once thrilled at my "detached and objective" description of the world of surgery would not be thrilled at these self-revisions from the distance of over twenty-five years. This is not to mention how creepy I now felt to be violating an old moral injunction: *De mortuis nil nisi bonum*. Writing the manuscript felt like coming clean when Arthur was an anonymous figure in a text; now that he was named and funds were being raised in his honor, it felt like slandering the dead.

My final reaction, the one that animates this writing, was to exercise a C. Wright Millsian "sociological imagination," to make of my private troubles a public issue. To use the experience of having my work unblinded as an opportunity to make confidentiality and anonymity a topic for exploration rather than a background assumption sealed in silence. To do that fully, I need first to make clear what I and my informants thought I was doing when I observed them; how none of us could reasonably have anticipated what happened when a text finally appeared; and how this, then, had consequences none of us could have foreseen. All of this is to say, if my own experience is an indicator of general practice, we promise confidentiality and anonymity in a way that is virtually an unthinking reflex. In my case, talk about confidentiality and anonymity was incantatory: words said to assure access; words said without much thought about their meaning; words I thought necessary to get a foot in the door; words, which if left unsaid, might stop my study before it started. The doctrine of informed consent demands that we do better than mouthing verbal formulas without conviction when describing our projects to our informants. It demands that we describe the risks attendant upon publication, with a special emphasis on the risks that may follow when somewhere anonymous and generic becomes this place here and when somebody generically representative become this person by name.

What We All Thought Once

Once upon a time, when the world and I were young, I entered the walls of Pacific Hospital eager to earn my spurs as a field-worker. With what I thought was a splendid sensitivity to the world I was entering, I had transformed my typical graduate-student scruffiness into a parody of respectability—trading in jeans and tee shirt for my nicest dress bell-bottoms; cleanest double-knit, no-iron polyester shirt; and a garishly colored, wide paisley tie; my then long, curly hair was smashed down and flattened especially for the occasion. I was as unprepared for the task as a human being could be—I had never taken a course in medical sociology, had never taken a course in field methods, and did not have an adviser with anything but a cursory acquaintance with ethnographic methods.[2] In truth, I had not yet even written a research proposal (I would not have one until the fieldwork was halfway completed). I entered the field with only a vague notion of what I wanted to study and with no earthly idea about how to study it. I wanted to study error and its control. The fact that with so little to recommend me the surgeons at Pacific allowed me access to do research remains one of life's sweet mysteries.

Six years later, give or take a few months, *Forgive and Remember: Managing Medical Failure* appeared. Its initial reception was positive beyond my wildest expectations. Favorable reviews appeared in popular media such as the *Wall Street Journal*—this I am convinced did more to bring the book to the attention of physicians than anything else—and the *New Republic*; professional journals such as *Science* and the *Journal of the American Medical Association* seconded this praise[3]; kind words in the sociological journals soon followed[4]; and even bioethicists noted the work—"Ethics in the Trenches" was the headline of one review. The book was an artistic and commercial success, acclaimed by many as an instant classic.

I recount all this neither to experience ego gratification nor to engage in a bit of vainglorious nostalgia for those lost, last glory years of the Nixon-Ford presidency. Rather, I want to recapture some of the feeling of the beginning of this enterprise, something of how much of an unknown quantity I was to the surgeons at Pacific. They did not consent to being the subjects of *Forgive and Remember*. How could they? None of us knew then, at the beginning, who or what I would observe, how I would describe and then interpret these observations, what form—if any—publication would take, and finally whether, if and when publication in whatever form occurred, the text would find readers. My informants agreed only to allow an unproven, even if earnest, graduate student to gather the data for his dissertation. Neither they nor I had any reason to expect that they had agreed to anything else.

Truth be told, most of them did not even agree to that. The actual beginnings were much too informal to be spoken of as an agreement between my informants and me[5] or even to be spoken of in terms that imply any sort of compact or contract. I first began, at a surgeon's suggestion, by simply observing mortality and morbidity conferences. I found that, as a white male in a tie, I could quietly slip into the back of the auditorium, take a seat, jot notes on file cards, and no one would ever ask who I was or why I was there. After a month of this, I went to one of my advisers to complain about how little I was finding and to suggest I better start over somewhere else on some more fertile topic. However, as I talked, we both realized that my nothing really was something. It became clear that I needed to get onto the wards for daily observations.

I returned to the senior surgeon who first suggested observation of the mortality and morbidity conferences to negotiate entrée and access. The senior surgeon listened to my plans but declined to help beyond giving me the phone numbers of the two chief residents. Anything more, he suggested, would be the kiss of death: the residents would never trust me, they would always assume that I was simply a spy for attending faculty, and they would never be forthcoming. I was miffed. I had wanted the way for my coming more cleared than this. For a couple of weeks, I dawdled before I could screw my courage to the sticking post and call one of the two chief residents.

When I finally met with the chief resident, he was courteous, if somewhat amused that I would want to pursue such a quixotic project. He said that if I were game, I could start the following Monday with him. This would be a good time since a rotation was occurring and all the members of the team would be new. This sounded good to me, even if I did not yet know what a rotation was or who was on a team. Be there for rounds he said. I agreed and asked what time. He said six thirty Monday morning. I tried to look like I did not find this extraordinary.[6] He added one more piece of advice—it was a warning I followed, not fully aware of what good advice it would prove to be: "If you really want to learn about us, you will have to live like us. Be here when we're here, including call. If you're in for a penny, you have to be in for a pound. Otherwise, you won't see anything, you won't understand anything you do see."

On the way out, I asked if I needed any permission from the chief of surgery or the faculty on the team. He told me not to worry; he would take care of it. As he escorted me out, we stopped at a laundry closet. From the stacks of laundered white coats he took one, placed adhesive over the red-stitched name, handed it to me, and said, "When this gets dirty, put it in the laundry and take another one."[7]

So there I was that next Monday morning, a bleary-eyed field-worker beginning research that was not yet so well thought out. There was no complex round of negotiations with hospital administrators who did not know until they were asked to review the manuscript prior to publication that the study had even taken place.[8] None of the medical students, none of the residents I observed, none of the attending faculty were given the opportunity to give their informed consent. Nor were any of the patients whom I observed, since to them I was just another member of the team. In fact, the patients were never even aware that a study was going on.

None of this bothered me at the time for a number of reasons. First, I assumed that the medical staff could always vote with their feet. With not much sensitivity to how the power and authority of the chief resident may have coerced their cooperation, I simply assumed that students and residents who did not want to be observed would avoid me. One or two did, but most did not. Since the attendings were neither insecure about exercising their authority nor shy nor timid, if they did not want me around, well, I figured they would have no trouble saying so since they did not seem to have any difficulty expressing themselves on a wide variety of issues. Finally, I did not think about consent from the point of view of patients at all.[9] After all, I was not studying patients. I was studying doctors and their belief systems. Occasionally I would feel like the imposter I was, when the surgeons made me stand last in line to stare through a proctoscopy tube—how could I justify making this uncomfortable, undignified procedure last even a few seconds longer?—or when the surgeons made me rake an abdomen, feeling for the mass that I could never detect. But, at the end of the day, none of this troubled my sleep. I was generally just another pair of eyes. I did not see how I was doing anything that might make a bad situation worse. Nor did I think of the patients' fundamental right to be free from any unwanted intrusions, however gentle.

The second reason that I never thought about issues related to the informed consent of my subjects is embarrassing to recount. I was simply and totally unaware of any requirement for informed consent in ethnographic research. I was not aware of seeing any discussions of consent in any reports from the field that I had read. My advisers—who, remember, were not field-workers—never mentioned informed consent to me.[10] The chief resident I negotiated access with never suggested that others had to consent to be studied. I can still remember when I first stumbled across the concept of informed consent. The Baker team was on call and I was with them. Work was uncharacteristically slow; a monster blizzard had inhibited the ordinary urban mayhem that normally paraded through the emergency room on a Saturday night. So we all found ourselves with some much-appreciated, if unexpected, downtime on our hands. After some desultory conversation about the weather, about the humiliations of overly long apprenticeship, and about where we might otherwise prefer to be and what we all would like to be doing there, reading materials were pulled out. The residents leafed through the medical literature. Dutiful student that I was, I had brought along a relatively recent volume by Barber and his associates (1973) on informed consent in clinical research.

As I leafed through the pages, I was fascinated. Who knew? Surely here was a set of reforms that were much needed, long overdue, and worthy of praise. I read with a certain smug, self-righteous satisfaction—now the biomedical research community would be more accountable. And what a good thing that was; it was about time their feet were held to the fire. What I did not do was make any connection between the biomedical research and my own research. Here were requirements for physician-researchers. They had, so far as I could see then, no applicability to my research undertaking or me. This was not a connection I would make until years later. And only then when I was informed that a research grant I was submitting to NIH needed to be vetted through the university's institutional review board, which I then sat on.[11]

My Own Limited Ethical Awareness

All of this is, as I say, to recover for both the reader and myself just exactly how naive and unaware I was at the beginning of my research of any of the ethical obligations that surrounded fieldwork in the hospital or anywhere else. In fact, there was only one ethical obligation that I recognized: subjects needed to be assured that what they revealed would be kept confidential and anonymous. Of course, because I was unschooled as a field-worker, this was not an ethical obligation that I had been socialized to or had learned in any formal fashion. I had received no formal lessons nor had I heard any lectures on the dangers of revelation nor did I have in hand any manual, cookbook, or bible that set out a code of conduct for me to follow. Rather, this was an obligation I was able to infer from my reading of the ethnographic literature.

In particular, two writing conventions alerted me to my ethical obligations. The first was the form "acknowledgments" took. Authors, when conveying their gratitude to the multiple parties that aided the production of their work, listed their informants first or saved them for last, to signal their special place. Then, they always wrote some variation of the following formula: "*I owe the greatest debt of all to the inhabitants of fieldworkville; they were unfailingly courteous and helpful in putting up with my silly questions and often pointless intrusions, in steering me down the straight and narrow, and in allowing me access to the most private domains of their lives. I owe them much more than this anonymous thank you implies, but I did promise to preserve their privacy (all the while writing a book about them). So these feeble words will have to do. But my subjects, the little people I now leave behind as I pursue my dreams of academic glory, know who they are and how much they mean to me.*"

There is a second convention of ethnographic writing that also alerted me to the importance of confidentiality and anonymity. As even the most casual reader of ethnography cannot help but notice, names are changed. Places with names specific enough to locate them on a map have those names changed. Generally the new names that ethnographers supply are somewhat generic, universal-sounding appellations. The North End of Boston becomes Cornerville in Eastern City (Whyte 1943, 1955). Newburyport becomes Yankee City (Warner 1961). Muncie, Indiana, enters the literature as Middletown (Lynd and Lynd 1957). Even after we know that Middletown is Muncie, the sequel is still titled *Middletown Revisited*. This kind of naming and renaming, the preservation of the original fiction even when that fiction is shredded and everyone knows where Middletown is, speaks clearly to the place of confidentiality and anonymity in the convention of ethnographic writing.

The emperor's new clothes aspects of these naming practices are perhaps best seen in the history of William Foote Whyte's classic *Street Corner Society*. The location of this study has so long been known that Whyte's field site has long been a visiting place for sociological tours of Boston, sacred ground for those making an intellectual pilgrimage. Beyond that, in the fourth edition, Whyte revealed both the identity of some of his subjects and also what had happened to them with the passage of time. Finally, a special edition of the *Journal of Contemporary Ethnography* was dedicated to revisiting Whyte's old stomping grounds. In this edition, we had the unusual spectacle of a more contemporary researcher challenging observations of fifty years ago by reinterviewing original subjects or their family members, all the while assuming that today's memory was more accurate than yesterday's report (Boelen 1992); a defense of the original work by Whyte (1992) and one of his subjects, a minor figure in the original text (Orandella 1992); a reassertion of the original text's classic status (Vidich 1992); and two troubling meditations on the whole controversy that sound a note of doubt and despair about locating an obdurate empirical reality and that settle instead for a position that extends primacy to interpretation (Richardson 1992 and Denzin 1992).

If confidentiality and anonymity were once important to this piece of fieldwork, clearly they no longer are; or at least they are not so important that anyone—original author, subject, reinterpreter—bothers to preserve them any longer. My own reaction to the controversy was sadness—I now knew too much for the book to exercise the same mythic effect it once did. I did not want to know who "Doc" was or what became of him. I wanted him there in that book for me and for others like me for whom it was an inspiration, a model of what we might hope to do. Some might say this disenchantment of the ethnographic world is a good thing. But I am not so sure.

On Not Naming Names

So I entered the field with an appreciation for the importance of confidentiality and anonymity. This appreciation was deepened by my reading both of classics in the ethnographic tradition and of other, more obscure works that followed all the same conventions of providing generic, all-purpose names, which act more as labels than identifiers.[12] I was aware that even relative novices were able to decode these labels at least so far as place is concerned. In fact, there was a not-so-secret thrill in this decoding; it was an initiation into tribal secrets, part of being transformed from an outsider into an insider. I recognized one other obligation as well: I felt—at a time of intense debate about whether neutrality was a correct methodological stance—that I needed to provide as impartial a description of what I observed as possible. Somehow, and my concrete, articulated understandings of this were dim, I felt if I got what happened right then this was a protection to my informants should my attempts to provide confidentiality and anonymity fail. When my subjects told me something in confidence and then worried out loud to me that what was said behind closed doors would not only become public but be traceable to them, when I sat down to interview my informants at the end of the formal fieldwork, when my presence as an outsider created apprehensions because of what I had seen or heard, I reminded my informants and myself that any work I produced would preserve their confidentiality and anonymity. These reminders always seemed to calm individual and group anxieties. Perhaps that is an indicator of the sincerity and conviction with which I was able to say the words. Lord knows I believed them. I never questioned them, really, even though I knew Cornerville was the North End of Boston and, much closer to home, Ward F-Second was at Brigham and Women's (Fox 1959)—and if I had really cared I could have tracked down the actual identity of the physicians involved in that study. The fact that I never questioned my own ability to provide confidentiality and anonymity is probably a testament to the convenient and self-serving nature of belief systems, even for those who study the way belief systems are convenient and self-serving for others. After all, if I had acknowledged to myself or my subjects my inner doubts, I could not have so aggressively pursued what Weber in another context calls the inconvenient facts upon which any sociological discovery rests.

These doubts did not surface until I sat down to make sense of my field notes, to create text and arguments out of observations, to create coherence where there had been a Jamesian "bloomin', buzzin' confusion." Very early in the process, it became clear to me that some version of what I was writing was going to have a life outside the university microfilms library of dissertation titles. I had a book and I knew it. But this discovery cheered me at one level and frightened me at another. For now, where there had once been blithe promises, all I saw was insuperable difficulty. In converting a dissertation to a book, how does a graduate student keep confidential the university hospital and medical school where the study took place? Occam's razor suggests that the reader interested in unblinding the study could get to the truth quickly enough. Knowing this, confidentiality and anonymity seemed like a promise doomed to be broken as soon as the book appeared. Like all authors, I wanted to be read and appreciated and not just by fellow sociologists but by surgeons, by health policy experts, by medical educators, by medical students and residents, by those in the emerging fields of medical humanities, by legal scholars concerned with malpractice, and by undergraduates whom I hoped to impress in the same way Whyte and Liebow once impressed me. If I were entirely honest, it was hard to imagine any gentle reader whose company I would shun. The worm in this apple of a fantasy was this: the larger the readership, the larger the betrayal of confidentiality and anonymity.[13]

There were three decisions that I made while drafting *Forgive and Remember* that were self-conscious attempts to preserve confidentiality and anonymity. In addition, there was a fourth, trivial change that the chair of the Department of Surgery asked me to make; I had no reason to resist this change, and, even if I had wanted to exercise my authorial authority for some pointless principle, I was not structurally in a good position to clash with the chair.[14] First, I decided to subvert deliberately one of the established conventions—giving generic identifications that correctly identify region. Pacific Hospital is not on the West Coast. I chose the name because it was deliberately misleading. I did not pick it out of the air. A dedicated Latin student in high school, I was aware of the original meaning of pacific—peaceful. Since Pacific was anything but, the irony pleased me. I did not then, nor do I now, worry that this deliberate deception was improper.

The next thing I did to preserve confidentiality and anonymity was not mention where I received my graduate education in the author's description on the back book flap. This was not because I was ashamed to have received my training there. Quite the contrary, I was, and continue to be, proud to have participated in the life of that department. Today, from the remove of so many years, I am pleased when my work is cited as continuing, extending, updating, and modifying that department's tradition of firsthand observation, its tradition of workplace studies, and its tradition of exploring medical education.[15] This omission was, of course, limited in its effectiveness. Sociologists who read the acknowledgments could figure out from the advisers thanked where I did my graduate work. Nonsociologists would not. My feeling then was that in erecting a wall of confidentiality and anonymity, one proceeds a brick at a time. The acknowledgments thank people but do not place them in geographic space.

The final change that I made was to switch the gender of one of my subjects. This switch is the topic of a related paper on fieldwork methods and ethics (Chapter 10). There was one woman in the program. I felt that I had to make her a man. It did not occur to me to switch genders the other way to preserve confidentiality and anonymity. Perhaps I thought such a switch would strain credulity. Whether I was aware of the consequences of the change is a matter of some debate. My wife and a friend remember my discussing this with them. They recall that I was concerned about the way this would create silence on gender dynamics but that I felt I had no choice. Their recollections serve me better than my own do; I recall no such conversations. I just remember a fairly reflexive gender switch.

In addition, there was one last pathetic attempt to preserve confidentiality and anonymity—the trivial one requested by the chair of the Department of Surgery at Pacific. I had identified a visiting luminary as Dr. Daily but then gave a correct university affiliation. The chair asked that I change the properly identified institution to Eastern University to avoid any embarrassment to Pacific or Dr. Daily since he was sensitive about the comment being made about him. Even before word processing, the change was no problem: retype a line, get out the rubber cement and a scissors, and voila, a revision.

So, on the eve of publication I felt that through misidentification, deliberate deception, and omission I had done everything I could, and more than most others in my position would, to preserve the confidentiality and anonymity of Pacific Hospital and, more importantly and much more personally, of my informants, attending surgeons and residents alike. To a very large degree, I succeeded. A number of reviews identified the site of the study as a "West Coast surgical training program." One reviewer went so far as to claim that the program could only be Stanford's. During the first years when the text was finding an audience, I received between twelve and fifteen phone calls from surgeons who had bets with colleagues about which training program I observed. None of these callers guessed correctly, and I somewhat priggishly would only tell them that I was not at liberty to reveal which institution was or was not Pacific[16]. All I would say was that I had received many similar calls. All of this pleased and puzzled me. The pleasure came from the sense that all this misidentification by surgeons was surely an indicator of some sort of external validity. The puzzle for me was the calls themselves—more often than not, the callers were certain I had studied their institution. How could they think this? Didn't they realize that they would have noticed being the subjects of extended primary observation? I never found a satisfactory answer to what their certainty that I studied them meant.

Of course, my ruses to hide the identity of Pacific, for all their success, failed as well. The place where they failed most spectacularly was Pacific Hospital. To this day, the place *Forgive and Remember* moves most briskly off the shelves is the Pacific University bookstore. In addition, my subjects were no great respecters of their own confidentiality and anonymity. Arthur, for example, greatly identified with my description of him—he seemed flattered by the sheer amount of attention I gave him. The negative in the portrait—the descriptions of his arbitrary displays of authority, his affect storms, and his unblinking irrationality—did not bother him. He saw just the positive—his commitment to patient care, his slavish devotion to the task, his integrity, and his unflinching honesty even when admitting mistakes. He was proud of *Forgive and Remember*; it was his baby, and I was simply the medium through which he spoke.[17] The person I called Arthur became Arthur, literally. He would go to surgical conferences and tell anyone within earshot about the book about him. For years, we carried on a friendly correspondence and not once did he sign a letter or card anything other than Arthur. When these antics of Arthur's were reported to me, they irritated me, but they did not surprise me. He was, after all, a loose cannon, incapable of being reined in by anyone. This is what attracted me to him to begin with.

What did surprise me—and upon reflection what should not have—was the reception of the book at Pacific Hospital. Naive as I was, I really believed that I would be able to preserve the confidentiality and anonymity of my informants.[18] It never for a moment occurred to me that I would fail precisely at the place where the anonymity and confidentiality were most necessary.[19] Outsiders, even if they know where Pacific is, still cannot decode the individuals. And even if they can do that, that decoding has few consequences. The unblinding of the text does not, as Schutz is so fond of saying, "gear into the world." Beyond the guilty pleasure of seeing a professional rival get his or her comeuppance or the umbrage at having a friend treated poorly by some unknown, smart-ass sociologist, the world has not changed; consequences are minimal. But this is not so for those in the institution; this airing of dirty laundry, these statements about colleagues' behavior made behind their backs in the heat of the moment now made public cannot be recalled. They do gear into the world and, by doing so, change it. The unblinding of a study, then, has real consequences at a local level. It can poison the atmosphere of naive trust that makes work possible. It can make the world a less happy place. These are consequences or risks to being studied that I never discussed with my informants because I was unaware of them. Beyond that, it is not even clear how I would have informed them, what I would have said, whether they would have understood. In the rehearsal, all these risks seem so hypothetical, so remote, so unreal, and so like yet unlike the ordinary risks of social life more generally.

So Why Not Give Up the Ghost?

So if things are as I claim, what is my complaint? If no matter what precautions were taken, none would have protected confidentiality and anonymity within the circle at Pacific, if my own subjects went around identifying themselves, then why carry on so on the basis of a single revealing fundraising solicitation? Aren't I taking myself a bit too seriously here? Isn't the only real harm here the one to my pride—the fact that I was not consulted and had no say in the fundraising solicitation? What else, if anything, besides wounded pride is at stake here? I see three problems clearly and have one concrete recommendation that will not avoid these problems but simply forewarn subjects of these dangers. First, I have emphasized that ethnographers in presenting their results in textual form change place names to give a sense that somewhere specific could be anywhere. We do this, I argued, to protect confidentiality and anonymity. But it serves us in other ways as well. Most importantly, it generalizes our descriptions. It takes the observations of specific things said and done and makes them more universal. As sociologists, we are rarely interested in the specifics for their own sake.[20] The practices we use to create confidentiality and anonymity protect our informants but they serve us as well.

For example consider the difference between these two equally accurate descriptions: First, "In the heart of 'Eastern City' there is a slum district which is inhabited almost exclusively by Italian immigrants and their children. . . . Cornerville is only a few minutes' walk from fashionable High Street but the High Street inhabitant who takes that walk passes from the familiar to the unknown." This description is the first and last sentence of the opening paragraph to the introduction of the 1955 edition of *Street Corner Society* (Whyte 1955, xv). But suppose Whyte had written instead this second version: "In the North End of Boston, there is an Italian slum district. . . . This slum is not far from Beacon Hill but the Back Bay swell that . . . " My own sense is that something sociological is lost in the second description that is present in the first. The second does not simply evoke society in the abstract way the first does.

Now to this, I anticipate two different objections. The first is that I have shifted my ground—I started talking about ethical apples and I have moved to rhetorical oranges. The fact that generic names make for discourse that is more recognizably and more convincingly sociological is very different from saying that we should do this because it protects subjects. True enough, but it does not seem to me that we can do one without the other. They are linked—confidentiality and anonymity do protect subjects—and in so doing help produce accounts that are more general, more sociological. When we generalize through our naming procedures, we make more transparent the work of sociology. Nowhere is it written that the proper ethical course has to disadvantage the person who practices it. Pointing out here how our self-interest dovetails with those of our subjects simply provides another, additional reason to live up to our obligations.

The second objection is more serious. By making a fetish of confidentiality and anonymity, we do nothing so much as make it impossible for others to check on the veracity of our work; we escape the methodological standards applied to other sociological work. After all, our colleagues who do not do ethnography have to describe their samples, to identify atypical features of these samples, and to provide arguments that justify their theoretic generalizations. When we use anonymity and confidentiality as I suggest we do here, then we create the suspicion that we are doing nothing more than using an ethical argument to avoid a methodological obligation.

This objection has some force but it misapprehends the nature of ethnographic description. At the very least, we have an obligation to describe fully those features of our neighborhood, those identifying characteristics that lead us to believe that we can generalize from our research setting to some wider social world. At the same time such a description makes clear the limits of the wider social worlds to which we are generalizing. For example, when I studied Pacific, I specified that the surgical training program that I was studying was in a poor urban area, was associated with an elite academic medical center and university, and was highly regarded for its past achievements and present accomplishments. I still do not see what more a reader would need to know, what anything else would add to understanding, what benefits are provided by more specificity. To the argument, "But Pacific might be unique," I can only shrug in bewilderment. To me, that argument places the burden of proof in the wrong place. Here, I would only repeat Everett C. Hughes' old argument:

> I am suspicious of any method said to be the one and only. But among the methods I would recommend is the intensive, penetrating look with an imagination as lively and as sociological as it can be made. One of my basic assumptions is that if one quite clearly sees something happen once, it is almost certain to have happened again and again. The burden of proof is on those who claim a thing once seen is an exception; if they look hard, they may find it everywhere, although with some interesting differences in each case (Hughes 1970, ix).

There is a second reason to resist the temptation either to unblind our studies even when we think no immediate harm will result or to allow others—even institutions proud of their ethnographic notoriety—to unblind our work. Here I employ a sociological variant of Tinker Bell's argument that "every time a child says that he or she no longer believes in fairies, a fairy dies." Each time an ethnography is unmasked, promises of confidentiality and anonymity grow weaker. For the ethnographers of the future and the sensitive topics they may wish to pursue, we need a muscular sense of confidentiality and anonymity. Those who have been asked to contribute to the Dr. Arthur fund may think twice about being asked to be subjects of sociological studies themselves. When we are tempted to throw in the towel and give up the ghost—as Pacific gave up Arthur's—we need to remind ourselves that we are all part of a research community. Our individual decisions have consequences for that community.

Finally, there is a third reason to safeguard confidentiality and anonymity with all the force we can muster. We have made promises to individuals and we ought to honor them. In revealing which institution was Pacific and which surgeon was Arthur, the fundraisers vitiated all those individual promises that I made. Some of my subjects might not care. In fact, some may go to surgical meetings and say, as Arthur did, "That character in that book—it was me." It is hard to control that behavior. People say and reveal things all the time that we might prefer that they did not. Moments of bad judgment and indiscretion are not rare in social life. Nonetheless, some might prefer to have their involvement kept secret just as they thought it would be. For some, those years at Pacific were painful and disappointing. They may prefer to have that pain and those disappointments stay private. The field-worker—and the institution—should honor those feelings.

Those are my objections, not so succinctly stated, to Pacific using my words to raise money on Arthur's behalf. To make them more than just a screeching baying at the moon, let me add one recommendation. It is a simple one. In promising confidentiality and anonymity we need to provide a full informed consent. Elements of this consent need to include at a minimum the following: a statement that, at a local level, readers are often able to figure out who our subjects are no matter what we do; a statement that there may be both short- and long-term consequences in the workplace and that this is a foreseeable risk of being studied; and a statement that while *we* will not reveal where we did our work or who was involved, we cannot control all others.

References

Anderson, Elijah A. 1979. *A place on the corner.* Chicago: University of Chicago Press.

Barber, Bernard, John J. Lally, Julia Loughlin Makarushka, and Daniel Sullivan. 1973. *Research on human subjects: Problems of social control in medical experimentation.* New York: Russell Sage.

Becker, Howard, Blanche Geer, Everett C. Hughes, and Anselm Strauss. 1961. *Boys in white: Student culture in medical school.* Chicago: University of Chicago Press.

Bissinger, H. G. 1990. *Friday night lights: A town, a team and a dream.* Reading, Mass.: Addison-Wesley Publishing Co.

Boelen, W. A. Marianne. 1992. Street corner society: Cornerville revisited. *Journal of Contemporary Ethnography* 21:11–51.

Bosk, Charles L. 1992. *All God's mistakes: Genetic counseling in a pediatric hospital.* Chicago: University of Chicago Press.

Buford, William. 1993. *Among the thugs.* New York: Vintage Books.

Denzin, Norman. 1992. Whose Cornerville is it, anyway? *Journal of Contemporary Ethnography* 21:120–32.

Fox, Renee C. 1959. *Experiment perilous.* New York: Free Press.

Geertz, Clifford C. 1983. *Local knowledge: Further essays on interpretive anthropology.* New York: Basic Books.

Hughes, Everett C. 1971. *The sociological eye: Selected papers on work, self, and society.* Chicago: Aldine-Atherton.

Kornblum, William. 1974. *Blue collar community.* Chicago: University of Chicago Press.

Liebow, Elliot. 1967. *Talley's corner.* Boston: Little-Brown.

Lynd, Robert S., and Helen Lynd. 1957. *Middletown: A study in American culture.* San Diego: Harcourt Brace & Co.

Orandella, Angelo Ralph. 1992. Boelen may know Holland, Boelen may know Barzini, but Boelen 'doesn't know diddle about the North End!' *Journal of Contemporary Ethnography* 21:69–79.

Richardson, Laurel. 1992. Trash on the corner: Ethics and ethnography. *Journal of Contemporary Ethnography* 21:103–19.

Van Maanen, John. 1988. *Tales from the field: On writing ethnography.* Chicago: University of Chicago Press.

Vidich, Arthur. 1992. Boston's North End: An American epic. *Journal of Contemporary Ethnography* 21:80–102.

Warner, W. Lloyd. 1959. *The living and the dead: A study of the symbolic life of Americans.* New Haven: Yale University Press.

Whyte, William F. 1992. In defense of street corner society. *Journal of Contemporary Ethnography* 21:52–68.

———. 1955. *Street corner society.* Chicago: University of Chicago Press.

Notes

1. Note even now that the institution has revealed that it is Pacific and that Dr. Somebody Specific, now dead and being honored, is Dr. Arthur, I do not feel free to be equally candid. They may have breached our agreement. That fact does not permit me to do the same. Strictly speaking, I suppose we could split hairs a bit. I made a promise to the institution to honor confidentiality

and anonymity. It did not promise to me that it would do the same. So it was free to do what it did. It certainly did not need my permission. Yet, I wish the institution had asked. I had made a promise both to the institution and to individual informants. The institution's behavior here has consequences for all those promises that I had made to individual informants.

2. I mean this to describe my advisers' state of knowledge as they and I saw it at the time. Truth is they gave wonderful advice whenever I found myself in over my head in dealing with my informants, they provided encouragement whenever I was down or overwhelmed by the human misery I was observing, and whenever they sent me back to the writing table, it was always with concrete suggestions that improved my work. I am still grateful—especially now that I have a fairly large catalog of horror stories from colleagues who were not so fortunate and now that I realize how difficult it is to provide useful advice.

   I should add that, unlike much of my behavior while in graduate school, my reasons for not taking a course in field methods had nothing to do with a late adolescent resistance to authority. Quite simply—and this was an indicator of the esteem with which ethnography was then viewed—my department had no one to staff the course. When, after my fieldwork was concluded, a new hire offered a course in fieldwork methods, I took it, even though I had long ago completed my coursework requirements.

3. The praise from medical quarters was not universal. One reviewer said that he could not escape the feeling that a "third rate intelligence" was making judgments on the "first rate." The reviewer for the *British Medical Journal* had trouble with my "over-decorated, jargon-ridden prose" although he allowed it was a common failing of "mid-Atlantic sociologists." He then asked, "Do we want to have such interpretative exposés when their theoretical basis is so slim, if not actually misguided?"

4. Like the medical reviews the reactions of sociologists were not universally positive. In the opinion of some, I had failed to see through hegemonic structures, had failed to see the structural arrangements that sustain cultural power, and was a mere apologist for the status quo. One or two reviewers attacked me for being a "neo-functionalist." I did not know what this meant, but it sure did not sound like praise in the context.

5. In my experience, my accounts of my methods have an orderliness and rationality on the page that they appear to lack in the experience. I do think this is a characteristic my work shares with all others in its genre. Part of this has to do with the didactic purposes of the methodological appendixes—we present them as lessons learned, pitfalls to be avoided, and recipes and tricks of the trade to be practiced. Part of this has to do with the rhetorical purposes of methodological appendixes—we present them as statements to assure skeptical readers that we gathered our data in ways structured enough to make what we have to say believable. Finally, part of this has to do with the ordering nature of words—when a torrent of experience is reduced to a trickle of words, a lot of what was accidental, contingent, or going on somewhere in the background gets washed away. It is this overly ordered sense of things that I have always suspected that Geertz is speaking of when he refers

to ethnography as a "fictio," a made or fashioned product. Ethnography, as well as descriptions of how it is achieved, describes social life; neither should be confused with the thing itself.

6. I did find it extraordinary. Up until this point, my course selection was governed by one simple rule—no matter how interesting, nothing before ten thirty. It seemed that course work completed, I was now throwing my lot in with folks whose biological time clocks were in a different zone than my own.

7. There is now, I realize, a debate about whether people like me should don white coats. Is it an unreasonable deception? Does it signal going too native? I did not think anything of it at the time. I would probably do the same thing again—I would just not have the luxury of being so unthinking. Over time, the coat began to have a talismanic quality for me. It reminded me of my distance from all those desperately ill patients whom I observed and, in a burst of magical thinking, I felt it kept that illness away from me. I did worry that walking through the halls someone who lacked a white coat's magical protection would collapse in front of me. And, as a result, I would be unmasked as a fraud. This far-fetched, fantastic fear remained just that.

I was always shy about going, unauthorized, into that linen closet and stealing coats as I needed them. What often happened was that when my coat got so ratty that it was an embarrassment to the team, one of my informants would march me to the closet for a replacement.

8. Lest this prepublication review sound like I recognized and was responding to some ethical imperative, let the reader be aware that this was not the case. This is what happened: while scanning the standard prepublication contract, I noticed that all legal liability from any statements in the text was assigned to me. Nervous about this, aware that I was revealing behavior that revealed in other contexts might be the cause for litigation—and this in the midst of a national malpractice crisis—I became alarmed and suggested to my editor that we ought to have some sort of review from Pacific Hospital to assure that the incidents reported were sufficiently veiled to preserve confidentiality and anonymity. Had I not reviewed the contract, I would never have asked.

To make an already long story shorter, the hospital attorney who reviewed the text thought everything was in order. He even wrote me a nice letter saying he enjoyed the text and that, from his point of view, it might even have a salutary effect by making clear how difficult a surgeon's life and work is. It was, of course, sentiments like this that caused those sociological reviewers of the earlier footnote to complain that I had become a dupe to those in power. But since their reviews were not in yet, I was pleased.

9. Let me hedge this ever so slightly. I thought a lot about consent of patients in their dealings with surgeons, particularly, and physicians, more generally. I wondered and fretted about how well they knew what was being done to them and why by their doctors. In the beginning of the research, I spent a lot of my time tagging along with residents as they got patients to sign their releases for surgery. I spent a lot of idle time marveling that surgery, which seemed so momentous to me, was treated so casually by doctors and patients.

10. The whole issue of ethical dilemmas in fieldwork—and my sensitivity to them—in fact became a sore point between my closest adviser and me. I would schedule appointments to confess some transgression that I thought I had committed or to get advice on some problem in which I was uncertain what the "right" thing to do was. He would talk with me. He would give me advice. But one part of that advice was always, "Remember you're not studying for the Rabbinate, you're a sociologist." I would, of course, get frustrated because he did not understand. He was, of course, frustrated that I was wasting his time with such trivial matters when there was so much serious sociology to be done.

11. And when informed of this, my first response was outrage. This was preposterous. What harm could occur as a result of this research? Where were the risks? And anyway, how could I interrupt the ongoing flow of interaction to gather consent each time a new participant entered the scene?

    Now, with all the zealotry of the newly converted, I worry my students to death about consent in their projects. Still, even with the best of intentions, in ethnography informed consent is easier to state as a goal than to achieve as a result.

12. I can think of works I read that identified a specific locale by name (Becker, Geer, Hughes, and Strauss 1961; Suttles 1966; Liebow 1967; Kornblum 1974; and Anderson 1979) but even here informants are assigned pseudonyms. Specificity is limited.

    Conventions are somewhat different in anthropology: where the fieldwork was done matters more. Even here informants are named generically. Yet the frequent inclusion of photographs—see, I really was there, it looked like this—in anthropological ethnographies undercuts some of the generality of pseudonyms. Of course, the chances that any of us actually knows that Truk villager, that Berber tribesman, that Yanamomo woman, are remote.

13. Before publication, I worried my informants with many questions but I never worried them with this one: Do you mind if your confidentiality and anonymity is breached? Maybe I did not want to know. Maybe the answer seemed so obvious that asking the question was unnecessary. Certainly, the chair of surgery, after reviewing the manuscript, made it crystal clear to me that a successful disguise of the institution and of the persons in it was important to him. I supposed he spoke for the whole. My discussions with him prior to the submission of the manuscript to the University of Chicago Press sobered and terrified me. It also, as I will describe in the text, inspired new flights of ingenuity to make the promise of confidentiality and anonymity more real.

14. Too many years later, immediately prior to the publication of *All God's Mistakes: Genetic Counseling in a Pediatric Hospital* (Bosk 1992), one of the genetic counselors went ballistic over the identifying name chosen to designate them. This informant felt that the name I chose—which had an ethnicity (and for that matter, a gender)—did not sufficiently veil this informant's identity. As a result, the informant felt that publication would damage professional reputation and standing (See Chapter 8). I thought my informant—and once upon a time friend and colleague—had it wrong. The fact was, genetic counseling was such a small world that little would prevent

the subject from being unblinded. I thought the name I had chosen worked at some un- or preconscious level to make group dynamics clearer. I also recognized that my being right had little or nothing to do with whatever resolution this conflict would have. I had promised subjects confidentiality and anonymity. I then felt I had to do whatever subjects asked to make this promise real. How reasonable I thought the request, or the grounds for it, was irrelevant. All that mattered was that the subject (informant) felt protected. That was what I had promised. In this case, the dispute was resolved when the informant was allowed to choose a pseudonym. The only restriction here was imposed by my editor who was worrying about production costs—the new name had to have the same number of letters as the rejected pseudonym.

As an aside to this aside, after I went over this episode in a fieldwork methods course, two of my graduate students who were conducting interview studies reported that during the informational preamble to their interviews when they covered confidentiality and anonymity, they asked informants to choose their own pseudonyms. They reported that this technique was a terrific icebreaker, that once interview subjects renamed themselves they engaged in wonderfully self-revelatory talk to explain their choice, and that the "feel" of these interviews was better than earlier ones before they adopted this tactic.

15. I may seem to be cute by not specifically naming that department here, but while it is certainly no secret where I received my degree, somehow simply saying so here in print would undermine the seriousness with which I am trying to treat confidentiality and anonymity in this paper.

16. Even today this misidentification continues. Now that I have been at the University of Pennsylvania for all of my postgraduate life, I am surprised at the number of physicians and sociologists who assume I did this work at the Hospital of the University of Pennsylvania (HUP), which was not likely since I had never set foot in Philadelphia until long after the fieldwork was completed. Recently, a HUP surgical resident visited me. He wanted to discuss *Forgive and Remember* but it was not the substance of the text that interested him. Rather, he had worked out which pseudonym went with which current member of the surgery department. I simply pointed out how long ago the work was done, how much turnover there is in academic departments. So even if he had been correct about HUP and Pacific being the same place—and I told him he was not—he would have been wrong about specific attributions.

17. This was an assessment that I continue to disagree with. It was, however, not an uncharacteristic judgment for Arthur to make. It was part of the narcissism, egoism, and self-involvement that I was straining, and if Arthur's reaction was typical, failing to describe. Knowing that I will have the last word here makes this harder rather than easier to write—remember, *De mortuis nil nisi bonum.*

18. It is late in the game to mention this but this paper wavered back and forth in naming those I studied *informants* or *subjects*. For me, *subjects* seems too detached, impersonal, and coolly clinical to accurately describe the relationship, to reflect all the time we spent together. On the other hand, *informants*

is not quite right; it errs in the other direction—it is too chummy. It does not accurately reflect the boundaries and distance that I worked hard to maintain. Neither term is right but they are the only ones I have. I use them interchangeably, creating first one false impression and then the other.

19. This is, of course, not just my problem. I share it with all researchers whose "bounded ethnographic whole" is a literate, intellectual group. All of us who study the kind of people who are not going to be intimidated by the type of book that might become an undergraduate text or find its way to the remainder table at a local bookstore need to recognize that our subjects can read us.

20. I am often asked how ethnography differs from journalism. The question is always asked in a tone that drips with hostility; nonetheless, it is a serious question and deserves a thoughtful answer, one more nuanced than this footnote will provide. But my simplistic and formulaic answer has to do with placement of details and their use. More often than not in journalism, the details are important for their own sake—they are the story. Like the Bauhaus architect Mies van der Rohe, journalists sacralize the details. Sociological ethnographers need to get the details right but it is what we do with them that elevates description into sociological theory. Like in so many other descriptions of this intellectual work or that, there is these days considerable "genre blurring" between journalism and sociological ethnography (Geertz 1983)—journalists provide more analysis here, ethnographers, more details there. This is especially true when journalists provide book-length accounts of specific cultural practices. For two good examples see Buford's (1992) account of soccer hooligans, especially his theory of crowd violence with its masterful summary of Freud, Tarde, Le Bon, and Durkheim—he skipped McDougall, but it is a theoretical tour de force nonetheless; or see Bissinger's (1990) description of Texas high school football.

Professional Expertise and Moral Cowardice

COUNTERFEIT COURAGE AND THE NONCOMBATANT

One theme of this volume, the emergence of bioethics within a sociological framework, asks why this discipline is rising to prominence now, who may legitimately claim to be a bioethicist; in light of that claim, what one is entitled to do; and what standards of accountability apply to those who act as an institution's officially designated "ethics" expert. A second theme concerns the doing of qualitative inquiry into such questions. My own engagement with bioethicists and their concern with research ethics impelled me to think harder about the ethics of my own practices: What is informed consent and do I provide it? What does it mean to promise confidentiality and anonymity and have so little control over whether that promise will be kept? Do we—and we certainly have reason to—underestimate the harms that may flow from being a research subject in a piece of ethnographic reporting while we overestimate the benefits? A recurrent question and tension connecting the two major themes of this volume has been: What is the proper relationship between social science and normative inquiry on medical practice?

Of course, I am neither the first nor the only person to ask this question, to experience this tension. In the last years of the 1990s, I participated in a number of groups and panels that sought to answer the question and resolve the tension. All of these efforts both succeeded and failed. The successes were predictable: questions were sharpened, dialogue was lively, and interdisciplinary networks were expanded. The failures were equally inevitable:

there were no definitive resolutions to any questions; tensions were as likely to be deepened as they were to be ameliorated. We might think of the problem of the proper relations of social science and moral philosophy, whether in medicine or in any other domain, as a hard problem, one that inheres in the nature of the domain, one that is unlikely to yield any permanent or, for that matter, satisfactory solution.

As an illustrative example, allow me to cite a call to a conference for which I presented a paper. The title of the conference was the politically provocative "Whose Ethic? Whose Medicine? The Tacit and Explicit Development of a Medical Ethic." The aim of the meeting, as stated in the conference brochure, was to provide a forum for discussing a set of questions. First, where does medical ethics come from? Is there an implicit and tacit ethic to medicine? If so, do ethics vary according to profession and specialty? Next, who knows medical ethics? Is it the province of a particular kind of professional or type of person? Or is biomedical ethics a matter of common sense or common knowledge? This was a conference to discuss a jurisdictional dispute among adjacent occupational groups (Abbott 1988). Once the "turf" question was settled, the conference was to move on to the even more slippery question of what a person with a legitimate claim to being an expert in medical ethics might do on that account. These questions were all for the first day.

On the second and concluding day of the conference, the brochure promised both a reflection on the accomplishments of bioethics over the last thirty years and an identification of some new problems that these accomplishments brought into view. The conference brochure, which I received long after I had agreed to be a speaker but before I had begun to prepare my talk, identified a variety of disciplines from which the experts who would highlight past achievements and predict future difficulties were to be drawn. I could not help but notice that my own discipline, sociology, was conspicuously absent from the list of fields that have contributed to the success, such as it is, of bioethics. This slight, unintentional as I am sure it was, nonetheless irked me as I began to prepare my talk on where medical ethics come from. As I set about writing my talk I decided to give a punchy, albeit disciplinarily dogmatic, gently self-deprecating, humorous homily that baldly asserted that all morality finds its origin in the structures of social life, is both externalized and internalized, is variable according to context, and that the time had come for different, sharper questions. Although I would have preferred to appear open-minded as I gave my talk, my training as a sociologist compelled a certain dogmatism with regard to the interdependence of ethics—all mental products, if truth be told—and social practice. This for me was a first principle of social science.

This was so despite the enormous diversity among the social sciences. Within my own university, the departments classified as being social sciences are various—anthropology, criminology, economics, history, history and sociology of science, political science, and sociology. The set of research methods—radiocarbon dating, statistical modeling, first-hand observation, focus groups, archival analysis, in-depth interviewing, random and targeted surveying, secondary analysis of aggregated datasets, content analysis of cultural products—when crossed by discipline then again by empirical topic creates so much variety that one can claim, with the same veracity, that like snowflakes, fingerprints, and karyotypes, no two social scientists are identical. In fact, so different are social sciences one from the other and each from all, that agreement and accord within and between departments is rare and prized. My colleagues in the divisions of natural science and humanities report that things are not so different in their respective camps; but, while this might be so, my talk was to concentrate on the intellectual terrain that I knew best—the border between sociology and bioethics.

So, despite the variation among social scientists, on the question I was asked to discuss—Where does medical ethics come from?—I thought there was something like unanimity. All social scientists agree—ethics come from the social. Despite its external origins, all social scientists would also agree that the type of human behavior that we characterize as self-consciously "ethical" also has an internal component. We surely disagree on how this internal component is formed; what significance it has for action; how easily it is changed; which methods are acceptable to accomplish change; and what part is hardwired, biologically programmed, or genetically determined, impervious to change given current technologies. Then, if we social scientists allow ourselves to bracket for a moment our disagreements about the nature, malleability, and importance of internal experience, once again we all quickly agree that ethics vary according to profession and specialty. Rights and responsibilities, duties and obligations, agency and relationships, core tasks and skill sets vary by profession and specialty, if only because social experience does so as well. Of course, we social scientists differ on how critical these influences are when compared to other sources of variation in ethical practice such as age, class, job title, gender, nationality, or religion.

So the first set of questions from the conference call tapped into my most dogmatic, pedantic voice, a screechy whine that I am better off not using but that I cannot seem to function without. So I wrote and imagined, while cringing, what I would sound like. Since Marx, Dewey, Durkheim, Freud, James, and Weber, there has been substantial agreement that we cannot meaningfully talk about ethics independently of the social situations in which ethical action is debated, defined, carried out, and questioned. Further, there is something in the social scientist that learns to distrust any actor claiming to possess or any action rationalized by either universal principles or unexplicated appeals to the collective good. As social scientists, we are taught to examine such statements so that we can find the self-interest that is cloaked in noble rhetoric. We are taught—and we continue to believe—that self-interest is there to be found. In graduate school nothing so much attracted my teachers' attention, ire, and red pen as a sentence containing the grammatical form *ought, should,* or *must* plus a verb. I learned first to give up this grammatical structure, then, like a subject trapped in some elaborately bizarre socio-psycho-linguistic experiment, I stopped thinking in these terms altogether. It was as if I had developed an allergy to arguments framed in explicitly normative terms. So my first impulse, as I prepared my talk, was to deny that the first set of questions with which the conference was to deal were really problematic: ethics are social, they are both internalized and externalized, they vary by time and circumstance, and no reasonably sentient creature thinks otherwise.

The more I thought about this approach—the more that I conducted a Meadian "dramatic rehearsal in imagination" of this line of argument, the more uncomfortable I became.[1] I knew that dogmatic does not work well in conferences. This is not an audience-friendly presentational style that works as a stimulus for discussion. Wrapping myself too tightly in a disciplinary flag seemed a strategy aimed toward deepening disagreement, trenching, rather than first identifying, then bridging, however tentatively, the organizational, political, economic, cultural, and moral differences within the diverse collection of individuals from many disciplines who share a concern with the socially visible activity that we call bioethics.[2] Beyond that, I was aware that a dogmatic denial of the validity of the questions contained in the conference call concealed much more than it revealed. The certainty that sources of ethics are social, that we both internalize ethics and reference itexternally in a variety of cultural artifacts, and that ethics vary by social circumstance tells us nothing about the content of that social ethic, provides no tools for evaluating how that ethic operates or for working to change it in those places where it yields perverse results. I believe that this tinkering and change, after considered reflection, is a critical part of the bioethics agenda. After all, as Marx, the sociologist, once noted while commenting on Feuerbach, the philosopher and theologian, the point is not merely to understand the world, the point is to change it.

Aware as I was that the tinny whine of my most pedantic voice was not the most effective tone for facilitating a dialogue, I searched for another note to strike as I prepared my talk. But try as I might, I still found irresistible the intense desire to lecture at the sheer naivety of those organizing questions: Where do ethics come from? Is there an implicit and tacit dimension to ethics? Do ethics vary according to profession and specialty? The very fact that the conference organizers asked those questions in that way meant that a central part of the explicit and tacit knowledge of the social sciences had somehow not been communicated to the world of bioethics. My felt need to lecture grew out of a sense of frustration. As a sociologist, I had failed to carry some very basic intellectual baggage into the world of bioethics. A failure that meant that, as a participant in the community of bioethicists, I was now placed in the position of reinventing a perfectly serviceable wheel or of sounding like a public scold as I pointed out the neglected sociological literature on the conference's orienting questions. The only way I thought to do this half gracefully, well aware that half gracefully is a euphemism for clumsily, was to deliver the whining lecture in an abbreviated form and then to spend somewhat longer exploring how my training as a sociologist (and that of my colleagues, most especially my ethnographic ones) created the conditions that allowed for our almost collective noninvolvement in the world of bioethics and how that lack of involvement then promoted the neglect that created the frustration that led to the necessity to adopt a hectoring lecture style. The material under the first subheading is the short abbreviated screed. The material under the second subheading is an attempt to understand what responsibility social scientists have for their relative neglect in the world of bioethics.

The Sociology of Ethics: Neglected Studies from the Shop Floor

There is a large sociological literature on the ethics of medical practice that is quite routinely ignored by bioethicists.[3] This literature is not clearly labeled "about ethics"; rather, the ethics emerges from a consideration of how people engaged in medical work struggle to do the right thing in a very imperfect world that imposes some very real constraints. The ethical or normative dimensions of everyday practice are probably seen most clearly in studies of the occupational socialization of recruits in medical school and then in residency training. One persistent theme of studies of medical socialization is that one of the faculty's goals achieved in an educational environment of total immersion through a variety of pedagogic styles is to stamp on recruits a professional identity.[4] Students are not sheet metal. A countertheme in the same literature is the tactics students use to evade, refashion, or sustain minimal personal damage in the loosely structured, all-pervasive process of identity change.

The social dynamic and theoretic dialectic that animates the literature on the process of professional socialization is the tension between the faculty's message and the student's interpretation of it. This tension is one of those Hughesian "rough edges" of social life where the seams that stitch together social life into a coherent whole are imperfectly joined. Rough edges are good places to tug if the goal is to change the nature of the social fabric.

All of this back and forth ultimately is about the rights and responsibilities of the physician's role, how one ought to act as a doctor, what one is permitted to do, and what one is prohibited from doing. The literature concerns how a medical ethic is formed in interaction, how its lessons are explicitly and implicitly conveyed, and how much room exists for recruits to interpret this ethic according to their own lights.

This is an empirically rich literature. One convenient, if shallow, way of ordering it is to think of the phases of a career in the medical workplace developmentally, beginning with studies of medical (Merton, Reader, and Kendall 1957; Becker, Hughes, Geer, and Strauss 1961) and nursing students (Olesen and Chambers 1968; Simpson and Back 1979), moving to studies of residency training, and finishing with studies of specific work sites, the ethnography of practice settings. When we do this in the form of a partial list, we find accounts of how that activity known as ethics becomes visible or is obscured in the training of physicians in the specialties of clinical pathology (Bucher 1961), internal medicine (Mizrahi 1986), obstetrics and gynecology (Scully 1980), orthopedic surgery (Knafl and Burkett 1975), psychiatry (Light 1980), rotating internship (Miller 1970), and surgery (Bosk [1979] 2003; Milman 1976).

This literature itself has a dual quality: It is focused on the details of the specialized occupational community—its operating rules, values, and principles, its everyday actions and their interpretation. It is also focused on very general, recurring problems of medical work—uncertainty, human fallibility, and the inevitable limits of incomplete knowledge and healing techniques. Most of the studies mentioned above are ethnographic; the data for them are the incidents of commonplace activities in the medical settings. Because of this, they report on how ethics are both explicit and open as well as implicit and tacit. That is to say, ethnographies report events and inscribe structured silences. Studies are organized around such themes as how resident psychiatrists deal with the professional failure that successful suicide represents (Light 1972), how students relate to their cadavers (Hafferty 1991), how residents in internal medicine redefine their core task as "Getting Rid of Patients" (Mizrahi 1986), and how surgical residents learn to distinguish blameless from blameworthy error (Bosk [1979] 2003). When taken as a whole, the range of phenomena with clearly normative dimensions that is covered by the studies of the occupational socialization of doctors and nurses is quite stunning: training for uncertainty (Fox 1957; Atkinson 1984), detached concern (Fox, Lief, and Lief 1963; Daniels 1961), the oscillation of cynicism and idealism (Becker and Geer 1958), the sociological calendar of professional development (Light 1975), the social accounting for error, the organization of time in the hospital and its relation to a profession's status and the moral community formed by its members (Zerubavel 1979), balancing the demands of professional and personal life (Broadhead 1983; Grant and DuRose 1984), as well as the tensions between doctors and nurses over the proper definition of care.

In addition to the considerable literature on how young recruits are transformed from laypersons to physicians and nurses, there is also a rich literature on specific practice settings that emphasizes how an occupational or work group's special mission guides action and determines what is proper in specific situations of risky choice. For example, we have Renee C. Fox's forty-year chronicle of the transplant community. *Experiment Perilous* (Fox 1959), *The Courage to Fail* (Fox and Swazey 1974) and *Spare Parts* (Fox and Swazey 1992) are all worth reading on their own; but, when taken together, they provide a narrative on continuity and change in risky experimental procedures; the interlocking worlds of doctors, patients, their families, and the wider community; and our definitions of personhood, life, and death. These works also illustrate how the same basic values can justify a wide range of empirical practices: behaviors change radically while the values that support them appear constant. When we read our ethics against the anthropologist Margaret Lock's work on transplantation in Japan (2001), we gain a deeper appreciation for how this ethics to which we attribute a certain naturalness, universality, and objectivity—after all, it is the transparent "rightness" of our own belief system, the sense that it could not be otherwise, that gives it much of its compulsive force—is culture bound.

There is also a rich ethnographic literature on neonatal intensive care units—a literature that grew and developed alongside these units. This literature explores, among other things, the following aspects of neonatal care: the process of decision making when there is conflict between staff or among doctors, nurses, and patient families (Anspach 1992); physician management of uncertainty through deliberately fuzzy communications (Prince, Frader and Bosk 1981); staff delivery of bad news to parents (Bogdan, Brown, and Foster 1982); staff consideration of family issues (Frader and Bosk 1981); and the negative impact of NICU regional organization on parental decision making at the same time that unit policies celebrate that same parental authority as the normative ideal for delivery of services (Guillemin and Holmstron 1991).

There is more. Sociologists have looked at how staff's evaluation of a patient's moral character (as inferred from the initial presenting complaint) determines waiting time (Roth 1972). Sociologists have looked at how responsibility and service obligations are defined by consultant genetic counselors and how these professional definitions shrink the opportunity for patient autonomy in some situations and swell it in others (Bosk 1992). Finally to close what has been an extensive but very far from comprehensive list, a list intended only to illustrate the range of ethical topics empirical sociologists have explored, sociologists have begun to look at how "ethics" itself operates in the academic medical center—what does it mean to call a problem ethical, who has the right to do so, when and how is such labeling encouraged or avoided (See Part One of this volume, Chambliss 1995, Devries and Subeudi 1998, Hoffmaster 2001, and Zussman 1992) and on presidential commissions (Evans 2002).

In the face of an empirical literature that has been very selectively sampled here—I have largely ignored the work of my colleagues in anthropology, folklore, history, political science, religious studies, and law; of my colleagues who look more closely at ethical issues from the patient's point of view (Frank 1996 and Charmaz 1991 are two richly textured examples); and of my colleagues in sociology who approach ethical questions with other than ethnographic research tools (see Christakis 1991 for an attempt to discuss ethics sociologically using a survey methodology that resembles the controlled clinical trial. Crane 1975 is an interesting early example; see also Barber et al. 1972 and Gray 1975 for pioneering attempts to use survey research data.)—I think we can understand how a sociologist who has spent the last twenty or so years of his career researching and writing about the everyday life of ethics in medical practice might take some umbrage at a conference call that neglected to mention sociology as one field among the many that have made a contribution to the study of medical ethics. With regard to medicine and ethics, we have a rich literature that demonstrates how ethics are social; how ethics are and are not taught by faculty; how ethics are and are not internalized by students; how ethical principles are codified in professional and organizational codes and rules; how these codifications are both imperfect, conflicting, and essentially incomplete and also frequently breached;[5] how ethical principles vary by a professional group's definition of its core task, its special mission, its shared identity and fate, and its core constituency; and how ethics are modified as a result of technological, political, organizational, or cultural change.

Of course, if I were somewhat more self-critical, I would both take less umbrage at the organizer's brochure and be more aware that I have severely overstated the sociological consensus on ethics, in general, or medical ethics, in particular. True enough, there has been, since Durkheim, something like agreement that ethics are social with an internal and external aspect. But to stop there is to pretend too much unanimity among social scientists. For although we agree ethics is social, we agree on little else. A number of points of view contend on precisely how medical ethics derives from the social and whose ends are served by professional ethics. Are ethical codes the expression of a service ethic that protect patients from exploitation? Or are they self-serving platitudes observed mainly in the breach that further the economic self-interest of the group that promulgates them? Do ethics guide action in situations of risky choice? Or do people act in ways that respond to exigent situational contingencies and then later rationalize those actions in terms of ethical principles that are elastic enough to be stretched to fit the situation? These types of questions remind us that agreements about the social nature of ethics are not identical to agreement about the nature, content, and social uses of ethics.

But I am not sufficiently self-critical to recognize these problems, and even if I were, I am much more interested in castigating the bioethics community for not recognizing the work of social scientists on how ethics operates in the everyday world of medical practice. In the normal course of this scolding, I am now obligated to recite the reasons that philosophers in bioethics are not sufficiently attuned to the empirical work of social scientists on ethical matters. The structure of this complaint is probably so well known that it is most likely as tiresome for those bioethicists who continue to read it as it is for me to repeat it here. Taking the form of a tedious litany, the scolding goes as follows: those concerned with medical ethics are too influenced by Anglo-American philosophy and too distant from continental trends that have a more phenomenological or existential bent. As a consequence, too

much concern is given over to a fruitless attempt to derive foundational principles that will apply universally. An excessive concern with the defense or
refutation of this principlism has retarded the growth of other intellectual
options. It has inhibited, as well, any genuine appreciation of the logic and
wisdom of cultural and ethical systems that place less value on the individual
than does American civil religion (Bellah 1970; see also Slater 1970, Bellah,
Madsden, Tipton, and Swidler 1985, and Putnam 2000).

In addition, the view of ethical problems championed at least implicitly
by many medical ethicists is empirically simplistic—it relies on individual
decision makers and decisive moments of action. Such a view is out of step
with how ethical problems develop over time; with the number of parties
actually involved and with the often divergent interests of those parties; and
with how decisions are actually made, questioned, re-evaluated, and revised.
Not only is the view of ethical problems in bioethics empirically naive, it is
overly restrictive as well. It is as if there were only two paradigmatic bioethics problems. The first involves a clinical problem at the bedside involving
a single patient: Do we initiate treatment? Do we withdraw treatment? Is
treatment futile? What does the patient want? Does the patient understand
the implications of wanting this? And so on. The second involves hypothetical conjecture around some new technological development: Is cloning
permissible? Who then should we clone? Who should pay? Other kinds of
problems are often ignored or labeled as social, economic, or political, as if
on that account, they cannot be ethical as well.[6] Hence, care at the end of life
is a problem that has worried bioethicists endlessly but the marketing practices of health care organizations receive little comment. Informed consent
for individual patients is an ethical problem, the algorithms organizations
use to determine treatments are not; they are viewed as trade secrets even
though they can properly be seen as an issue of informed consent.

The next move in the scolding is to point out that this limited view of what
an ethical problem is and how it is solved is one that allows the bioethicist to
work closely with physicians without challenging the prevailing structural
arrangements of health care.[7] In this critique, the success of bioethics indexes nothing so much as the failure of bioethicists to ask tough questions,
to champion structural reform, or to threaten entrenched organizational
interests. Bioethicists, who like to discuss how the coming of ethics to medicine has transformed the doctor-patient relationship, do not take kindly to
this last criticism, which is, in truth, not entirely fair.[8]

The problem with this criticism, other than that it has become tendentious having been made so many times before, is that it is too one-sided in its

allocation of blame. Bioethicists have ignored useful social science perspectives and research; and we social scientists argue that this is only because of the intellectual shortcomings of philosophers. This critique, locating as it does the problem in the individual failings of philosophers rather than in the structural situations in which knowledge is created, disseminated, acknowledged, rewarded, or ignored is surprisingly unsociological. I do not know of any discussion by a social scientist that flips the perspective and asks, What are the problems with social science, or social scientists, that it, or they, cannot adapt to the new world of medical ethics and make it, or themselves, useful? I often wonder if the unattractive bitterness that I detect in my critique and that of my colleagues is not some form of Schelerian *ressentiment* (Bershady 1992), an ill-disguised form of "sour grapes." After all, before there was bioethics and bioethicists in the academic medical center, there was social and community medicine, behavioral medicine, and social scientists. In the zero-sum game that is medical school curriculum time, or attention in public arenas (Hilgartner and Bosk 1988), as ethics has waxed, social science has waned. In the last section of this conclusion, I stop scolding medical ethics for its inattention to social science research and ask instead what inhibits social scientists from taking a more public role in the world of bioethics. I ask what is the social scientist's problem: How is it that we can research topics of direct relevance to the questions that bioethicists are interested in and do it in such a way that not only is that relevance not apparent to those involved in medical ethics, but it is also actively disavowed by social scientists when the work is noticed by medical ethicists or makes its way into the public arena? We social scientists have been so intent on demonstrating how we are different from bioethicists that we have not given enough consideration to what similarities might mean.

The Professional Outsider

C. Wright Mills (1959) defined the sociological imagination with a wonderfully evocative aphorism as the ability to see in personal troubles, public issues. By this, he meant to suggest nothing more than that few of our troubles are uniquely our own. Rather, our problems, like our values, our criteria for choosing among courses of action, and our standards for evaluating that action are all socially structured. Following Mills, I assume that my frustration with bioethicists (and to be fair their frustration with this sort of carping from me) is not unique to me, merely or only a private trouble, it is also socially structured and hence capable of becoming a public issue.

This transformation from private trouble to public issue is the work of the remainder of this conclusion. Let me start by returning to the simple question that was described in the introduction to this volume as an index of *angst*: "What would you do in this situation?" I still think of this question as one of the most terrifying private troubles that I can experience as a social scientist whenever I stumble from my ivory tower into the everyday world of medical practice, which now features ethical questions as a visible, and sometimes prominent, organized social activity. As I stated in the Introduction to the volume, this situation or trouble is one that repeats itself quite regularly when I am in the field doing research and, even more frequently, when I am doing some sort of outreach as a faculty member in the Department of Medical Ethics. I still do not know how to respond whenever a physician, nurse, or very occasionally, a patient turns to me in a conference room or even a private conversation and asks, "Well, what do you think I/we should do?"

A cavalier response like "ask an expert" is clearly wrong; it is hard to justify a wiseacre putdown of those in need of help. But beside, at the crudest level, knowing what not to do, I remain with nearly thirty years of experience at a complete and total loss. The moment remains a tense and anxious one for me. I still resist a direct answer while trying to sustain some pretense of graciousness; this charade of civility almost always fails, in my eyes at least, because of my inability to suppress my displeasure when asked this question: "Why can't these people learn that's not what I do, what's wrong with these doctors? I don't ask them to be bankers, why do they keep asking me to be an ethicist?" With patients, I have more patience but no greater desire to be forthcoming. As I mentioned before, sometimes my resistance fails either because I feel sympathy for people so at sea that I want to do something or because I feel trapped by situational exigencies into giving an opinion.[9] My generalized insistence on not answering, when they are asked, questions that require a normative answer is both principled and self-defeating. Such an outcome is not entirely unexpected since my own personal unwillingness to enter the discourse about what we should do right now is both bottomed on a number of questionable premises and undercuts any claims I might make about why letting me observe is important and useful.

Chief among the questionable premises on which my silence rests is this tortured syllogism:

Major Premise: Experts should answer only those questions where they have a specially trained competence. Sociologists are trained to answer empirical questions.

Minor Premise: What would you do is a normative *question.*

Conclusion: Because social scientists, in general, and ethnographic sociologists, in particular, are trained to answer empirical questions, they can claim no special competence in answering normative questions. Therefore, they should be unwilling to do so.

Normative questions to moral philosophers and theologians, empirical ones to the various social sciences make a limited amount of sense as a decision rule for the division of academic labor. Even here it is highly imperfect and difficult to apply. There are very few normative questions without an empirical component and very few empirical questions without a normative component. The decision rule describes the actual work of philosophers and social scientists quite poorly: what could be more anchored in the empirical world of scientific communities than Thomas Kuhn's (1970) discussion of the paradigm problems in normal science and the paradigm shifts of scientific revolutions? What could be more mindful of the normative world than Mary Douglas's (1966) discussion of social organization, and the threat to order that occurs when the sacred mixes with the profane? As a guide for practical action, a decision rule that allocates operational questions to social scientists, ethical questions to philosophers and theologians, and policy questions to management is a peculiar form of nonsense—an odd denial by sociological ethnographers of what everyone knows about how problems of medical ethics present themselves in the social space. Ethical problems index social and organizational troubles, perhaps even more vividly than they do normative ones.

For surely in the early years of bioethics when large medical decision-making dilemmas became visible as widely covered, instant cases rather than being treated as troubling private decisions, much more than a question of values was involved. Before we as a society evolved the operational solutions that we now utilize for resolving ethical conflicts, the way a private value conflict became a visible ethical problem was to be a troubled social situation. These were cases (Saikewicz, Brother Fox, Karen Anne Quinlan) where all the normal problem-solving strategies of the organization failed to provide a workable solution, where the normal course of illness failed to make a situation go away through recovery or demise, and where each party distrusted the other's capacity to discharge role responsibilities in good faith.[10] In these first public treatment crises, values were involved to be sure, but this was not some sterile intellectual debate between two sweet reasonable souls each intoxicated by the aesthetic pleasure of rational debate. The fact that sociologists had no difficulty recognizing or writing about the social character of ethical disputes but then were chary of taking any responsibility for discussing what should be done as the disaster unfolded strikes me now as an odd form of intellectual and moral cowardice. By the same token that moral philosophers with little to no experience at diagnosing social dynamics acted as if they were "moral engineers"[11] who could reason their way to an equitable outcome strikes me as hubris. This is so even though those moral philosophers had private moments of doubt that they did not share with those publics to whom they were trying to convince that they had something of value to offer:

> . . . Unfortunately, the role of professional (particularly the *paid* role) offers no special encouragement to indulge the gap between private agony and public sentiments. . . . One gets pushed, and tacitly approves the pushing, to stay away from the dark corners of doubt and uncertainty, of deeply felt inadequacy. One is asked to bring light, lucidity, and logic, and one is only too happy to accommodate the request. They don't want a dolt, a muttering victim of private struggles with darkness and ignorance; they want a pro. . . . (Callahan quoted in Stevens 2000, 55, emphasis in original).

Even those clinical bioethicists whose ambitions were less grand than Callahan's, those who did not define their task as pronouncing the ethically correct solution to otherwise intractable problems but rather saw their task as facilitating a discussion, opening a conversational space, or structuring an equitable process, even they were guilty of considerable social naivety as well as hubris. To be fair, without this naivety about the complexity of the social situation and without this hubris about the efficacy of reasoning from principles, deficiencies in then-current practices might have never been confronted.

This pattern of withdrawal by social scientists and engagement by philosophers continues into the present. The ethics functions in health care have become specialized, professionalized, internalized and bureaucratized in health care organizations; new occupational roles with specialized training and career ladders have emerged, new regulatory structures with new reporting structures have been created, and private decisions have now become public matters. Despite organizational and cultural changes of enormous magnitude, these phenomena have received precious little commentary from social scientists. This lack of interest is itself peculiar. One would think that from the point of view of social movement theory or the theory of professions, the emergence of the professional ethics expert within organizations would excite great research interest. Beyond that, the emergence of the bioethicist presents interesting puzzles for organizational theory. After all, any attempt to make client autonomy a basic operating principle in a bureaucratic organization is very quickly going to be involved in some interesting empirical paradoxes. How removed social scientists can be from resolving these paradoxes, as health care organizations seek to confront them, is an open question. While our distance is said to cultivate objectivity, at the same time does it not remove some of our legitimacy as organizational, social, or practical experts?

I suppose that if I were accusing of moral cowardice anyone other than myself and my closest colleagues, who, like me, get all twittery when it is suggested that our research forces upon us difficult normative choices, I might have to provide more evidence than I do here of such a strong charge. Here all I wish to add as additional support is an expanded impressionistic discussion of data already reported. I am not alone. Every ethnographer who works in medical settings that I have ever asked admits that being asked, "What would you do?" is terrifying. All report trying to evade giving a direct response. All report that their first response to being asked a normative question is, "Can we study it some more?" And all report a certain reluctance to be involved in everyday practical ethics. Perhaps calling this stance moral cowardice is too harsh; perhaps this is nothing more than intellectual prudence, an honest recognition of the limits of the tools of our trade. While this may be so, still it is hard to make something noble out of collective avoidance of the question, "Well, what would you do?" The gentlest revision of my charge that I am willing to make is that we ethnographers display a fully informed, voluntary moral cowardice. We are aware of the risks and benefits of this course of action and choose it over other available alternatives.

This moral cowardice is informed first of all by the accidental nature of our expertise. Until recently, none of us set out to study explicitly the normative dimensions of medical practice. Rather, these dimensions of practice came into view as we tried to discover other aspects of the everyday world of doctors. Having received intense training in the necessity of avoiding moral judgments, especially of the sort that would privilege one set of beliefs over another, any request for just this sort of judgment seems outrageously illegitimate. So, a good portion of our informed moral cowardice grows out of a disciplinary discomfort with normative questions. Another portion of it grows out of the ways we are taught to think about empirical questions once we bracket the normative aspects, which we are free to discuss and analyze so long as we do not judge them, so long as we realize that the values that we are talking about are merely a "social construction," and so long as we recognize that if values were not organized this way, they would be organized in some other way and that other way would have problems of its own. An interesting feature of our training is that the more likely we are to find features of everyday normative judgment and action wanting, the more intensely we look for good reasons to explain it in a nondemonizing fashion, the more we resist making judgments about the way social life is organized here. But even if we were not taught to avoid normative judgments, we would still be at sea when asked, "What would you do in this case right now?"

We social scientists practice a generalizing craft. We are experts on what happens on average, generally, under the following conditions. Even those of us who do not use statistical methods are still taught to think in terms of central tendencies and normal variation, means and standard deviations, spurious correlation and sample bias. We are experts of the scatter plot, masters of the distribution. What we are not is expert at predicting where any point falls in the plot. The question "What would you do?" is not only normative, it also calls for just the kind of individual assessment that is quite outside our zones of competence. In fact, for a social scientist to pronounce on the instant case—to judge the individual and specific on the basis of group characteristics—is to commit the "ecological fallacy." And, well, we social scientists are all too well behaved to do that in public.

But, while this description of sociological reticence in the face of normative questions is accurate as far as it goes, it has a number of limitations. First, it ignores the considerable normative freight that much of the work in medical sociology carries. Freidson, Fox, Becker, Goffman, Parsons, Hughes— these are not sociologists whose writings on the medical profession contain no normative judgments. As a characterization of a response, it rests much too heavily on a pair of classic false distinctions: fact and value, empirical and normative. The pretense that they are separable when we know better is a way of avoiding the difficulties that decision and action require. Next, the reticence sociologists report when they are asked normative questions in clinical situations is described here in terms that are too cognitive, rational, and universal. This account excises the affective and self-interested aspects of at least this sociologist's reluctance to engage normative questions directly. To be completely candid, it is these last mentioned aspects that are more important to me than the academic reasons advanced so far, all of which have the character of a set of post hoc rationalizations. My aversion to answering normative questions directly arose long before I could articulate reasons for it.

The first time I experienced this aversion occurred long before I studied medical ethics, before I had ever heard the term bioethics, before I realized that I was a medical sociologist, and long before I had self-consciously thought about my role as researcher. I was three weeks into my fieldwork as I watched the chief resident get into an argument with a senior resident about the treatment of a patient—there was an ethical dimension to the argument since it involved how to present treatment options to a patient. This was long before anyone thought candor a good idea, only a few fringe types advocated anything like full disclosure—it was not really all that long ago. What started as an ordinary disagreement very quickly spiraled out of control. The sleep deprived, as I was soon to discover, have short fuses. Soon they were jaw to jaw, speaking in tones much louder than the distance required for each to be heard. Faces reddened, neck veins began to bulge and throb. It was very clear to me that neither was going to back down. I went into fly-on-the-wall mode, scrunching down in a corner on a stool, scribbling it all down furiously. Then without warning the chief resident wheeled around toward me and said, "Okay, Bosk, which of us is right? *What would you do?*"

It happened that at that moment I was asking myself the same question. And I truly did not know. It did not much matter that I could honestly admit to seeing both sides—the question still flustered me. I saw it as a threat. If I identified too clearly with one party, then the other might become angry.[12] Declaring myself, had I anything to declare, would skew the kind of data I was just beginning to gather. Not declaring myself carried the same danger. How was I to avoid unwanted, uncontrollable, unmeasurable observer effects? I was silent not for ethical reasons. If I had reasons they were pragmatic. Mostly, I was not quick enough to do anything but stammer. I became a joke—a figure too flustered to manage to speak. So, by appearing to be the clown, I defused the argument but not intentionally.

Over the years this example marks one paradigmatic situation for being asked, "What should we do? What would you do?" The first time this happened I had no earthly idea, no way to formulate an answer. But over the years this was not always so. In studying genetic counselors or neonatal intensive care, I was asked the questions when I had very strong opinions about what should be done and I demurred on those occasions as well. My own belief was that I was there to record what went on not to change it in the instant case. I truly believed that my sense of an answer, when I had a sense of an answer, was not based on specialized knowledge that I had as a sociologist or as an ethnographer. Answers such as those that I was unwilling to give at the time were informed by reasons, values, feelings, and considerations that I would call nonprofessional. They were not invalid on that account nor were they any less thoughtful—they were just not bottomed on what allowed me to be in the position to be asked these questions that I did not want to answer: namely, whatever skill I possess as an ethnographer of medicine.

There is a second situation in which I am now commonly asked for my opinion. This occurs at meetings that I attend at the medical center when others are aware that I am a faculty member in the Department of Medical Ethics. I am still reluctant to answer. But there the concern is less conditioned by pragmatic considerations like the future of a piece of research. In part, the reticence stems from a discomfort with being identified as a bioethicist. At these times I want to scream: "*Look, it's a multidisciplinary field. All ethicists are not alike. I'm the kind of ethicist who doesn't answer ethical questions. I just study them so I can ask even sharper questions later.*" My reticence stems as well from a sense that the more directly I answer, the more directly that I pretend to be the kind of ethics expert who has answers, the less able I am to act later as an ethnographer of medical ethics as it unfolds in this setting or that. The fact is, the more involved I am in any answer, the less I am detached. The more I advocate for this or that policy or course of action, the less able I am later to describe, analyze, and interpret the motives, interests, and purposes of the various parties in this setting or the next or the one after that.

Conclusion: Looking for Genuine Counterfeit Courage in the Noncombatant

In a much-cited paper, Mark Siegler (1979) argues that only physicians should be allowed to act as clinical ethicists. The rationalization for what otherwise looks like straightforward claiming of threatened occupational turf is simple: only physicians have been trained in the intricacies of the doctor-patient relationship, only physicians have the experience to talk sensitively to the vulnerable, only physicians can appreciate what is at stake in these discussions. Ignore for the moment the obvious counterargument: had physicians been adequately trained, were they able to talk sensitively, could they but appreciate what was at stake, there would never have been the need for bioethics and bioethicists to emerge. Pay attention instead to Siegler's worry and the language with which it is expressed. Siegler worries new strangers at the bedside will make matters worse because they will display "the counterfeit courage of the non-combatant." Clinical bioethicists will advocate a course of action for which they need not be accountable. A bad situation will be made worse.

Siegler's position did not win the day for a number of reasons. Two are worth mentioning here. First, to a large degree physicians troubled by their isolation from the community, by their own difficulty in talking through dilemmas with patients, and by their need to share decision making more broadly invited noncombatants into the hospital. Siegler was, in essence, trying to cancel the party after the invitations were issued and the responses returned. Second, a major part of the critique of medical practice by bioethicists and others concerned the dominant role of physicians and the way this role was used to usurp the personal autonomy of patients. Siegler's argument came after the time when some social consensus had been reached that medical ethics, as war for generals, was too important to be left to physicians. Here, it is perhaps necessary to add that in modern warfare, generals are noncombatants. Command centers are located far from actual battlefields.

Siegler lost the debate, such as it was, and has since admitted that perhaps he was wrong. Clinical ethicists have not roiled the waters with "the counterfeit courage of the noncombatant." I would argue that they have done something else. They have adopted medical styles, medical language, and medical roles (Chambers 1996). They fit right in. On many of the disputes on which their advice is sought—issues surrounding futility and treatment withdrawal—medical staff are deeply divided. Clinical ethicists mediate tensions that already existed within the organization. Beyond that, there is now some evidence that they help hospitals save costs by doing so (Schneiderman et al. 2003).

Siegler, it appears, had no reason to fear the "counterfeit courage of the noncombatant." With the benefit of hindsight, this seems obvious. Counterfeit courage is, first of all, often difficult to tell from the authentic kind. One way to be courageous is to appear or pretend to be courageous. This is, I would argue, exactly what clinical ethicists have done. Their role models have been those physicians and surgeons in critical care units, dealing with high-risk patients with multisystem problems who asked for their aid. As a result, the ability of clinical ethicists to challenge the status quo has been quite limited. Over time, "strangers at the bedside" have been assimilated to the team. How could it have been otherwise? In addition, Siegler's fears were baseless. Once invited into settings, clinical ethicists were no longer noncombatants. They were engaged. They had positions to defend, organizational turf to protect and expand—they had a mission, a constituency, and a putative set of skills.

With all this, I find myself in a curious position. I was a strong advocate for the kinds of conversation clinical ethicists are said to encourage before they happened with any frequency. In fact, I found myself expressing a substantial amount of outrage for someone trained to be nonjudgmental that such conversations were more observable in the breach than in the event. But now that those conversations take place in an organized fashion, according to bureaucratic procedures, led by people who claim a special competence, I find myself both profoundly skeptical and wishing for some genuine "counterfeit courage" among noncombatants. I find both in short supply.

I would take "genuine counterfeit courage" to be something like humility, some willingness to question what the enterprise of clinical ethics is about, who it serves, how it is organized, what its goals should be, and how it should be held accountable when, and if, it fails to meet its own expectations for acceptable performance. But, in the current climate, I do not think it reasonable or fair to expect bioethicists to do this. They need to convince too many other entrenched interests that they are valuable. They have to strive too hard not to appear the "dolt, a muttering victim of private struggles with darkness and ignorance . . . " as Callahan said. He was right when he insisted that what was wanted in this contested terrain is "a pro." Callahan also correctly identified that what was needed for continual progress of the bioethics project—if it was to be more than just another exercise in the claiming of professional turf—was highly contradictory.

> Somehow or other, as we become more professional, we will need to find ways to become less so. . . . The only way out is to keep returning to the discrepancy between how we tend to think about health and illness privately, late at night, and how we talk about them professionally. (Callahan in Stevens 2000, 56)

For this, I think, we need a noncombatant; that is, someone who is able to observe bioethics as it develops, but whose interests are not tied to its growth. It is not that bioethicists are incapable of "returning to the discrepancy between how we think privately, late at night, and how we talk professionally." But no professional group—ethnographers and social scientists included—should be entirely free to choose when to examine these discrepancies and which discrepancies to examine. Bioethics needs an other to confront its settled pieties, its smoothed-over discrepancies, the unresolved contradictions that become part of the way the world is. This figure need not be an ethnographer—representatives of advocacy groups can do this work as well (Chambers 1999).

But bioethics as it professionalizes, as it organizes, closes down some of the space that it once opened up. The enterprise retreats to its defensible borders, which may be quite extensive—this kind of scholarship, that kind of ethics consultations, and these sorts of public policy roles. As this happens, bioethics will need to find ways to remain open to skeptics, critics, and interested observers. And we, social scientists and ethnographers, will need to find ways to demonstrate that we can be useful without being helpful.

References

Abbot, Andrew. 1988. *The system of the professions: An essay on the division of expert labor.* Chicago: University of Chicago Press.

Anspach, Renee R. 1993. *Deciding who lives: Fateful choices in the intensive care nursery.* Berkeley: University of California Press.

Atkinson, Paul. 1984. Training for certainty. *Social Sciences and Medicine* 17:949–56.

Barber, Bernard, John J. Lally, Julia Loughlin Makarushka, and Daniel Sullivan. 1973. *Research on human subjects: Problems of social control in medical experimentation.* New York: Russell Sage.

Becker, Howard, Blanche Geer, Everett C. Hughes, and Anselm Strauss. 1961. *Boys in white: Student culture in medical school.* Chicago: University of Chicago Press.

Bellah, Robert. 1970. American civil religion. In *Beyond belief: Essays on religion in a post-traditional world.* New York: Harper and Row.

Bellah, Robert, Richard Madsden, William M. Sullivan, Ann Swidler, and Steven M. Tipton. 1985. *Habits of the heart: Individualism and commitment in American life.* California: University of California Press.

Bershady, Harold. 1992. *On feeling, knowing, and valuing: Selected writings of Max Scheler.* Chicago: University of Chicago Press.

Bogdan, Robert, Mary Alice Brown, and Susan Bannerman Foster. 1982. Be honest but not cruel: Staff/parent communication on a neonatal unit. *Human Organization* 41:6–16.

Bridge and Bridge. 1981. The lonesome life and death of Christopher Bridge. *The Hastings Center Report* .

Broadhead, Robert. 1983. *The private lives and professional identity of medical students.* New Brunswick, N.J.: Transaction Books.

Bucher, Rue. 1961. Conflicts and transformations of identity: A study of medical specialists. Ph.D. dissertation. University of Chicago.

Bosk, Charles L. 2003 [1979]. *Forgive and remember: Managing medical failure.* 2nd ed. Chicago: University of Chicago Press.

———. 1992. *All God's mistakes: Genetic counseling in a pediatric hospital.* Chicago: University of Chicago Press.

Caplan, Arthur. 1982. Ethical engineers need not apply: The state of applied ethics today. *Science, Technology & Human Values* 6:24–32.

Chambers, Tod. 1999. *The fiction of bioethics: Cases as literary texts.* New York and London: Routledge.

Chambliss, Daniel. F. 1996. *Beyond caring: Hospitals, nurses, and the social organization of ethics.* Chicago: University of Chicago Press.

Charmaz, Kathy. 1991. *Good days, bad days: The self in chronic illness and time.* New Brunswick: Rutgers University Press.

Christakis, Nicholas A. 1999. *Death foretold: Prophecy and prognosis in medical care.* Chicago: University of Chicago Press.

Crane, Diana. 1975. *The sanctity of social life.* New York: Russell Sage.

Daniels, Morris. 1961. Affect and its control in the intern. *American Journal of Sociology* 66:259–67.

DeVries, Raymond, and Janardan Subedi, eds. 1999. *Bioethics and society: Constructing the ethical enterprise.* Upper Saddle River, N.J.: Prentice Hall.

Douglas, Mary. 1966. *Purity and danger: An analysis of concepts of pollution and taboo.* London: Routledge and Keegan Paul.

Evans, John. 2002. *Playing God?: Human genetic engineering and the rationalization of the public bioethical debate.* Chicago: University of Chicago Press.

Fox, Renee C. 1957. Training for uncertainty. In *The student-physician,* ed. Robert K. Merton, George Reader, and Patricia Kendall. Cambridge, Ma.: Harvard University Press, 207–41.

———. 1959. *Experiment perilous.* New York: Free Press.

Fox, Renee C., Harold Lief, and Victor Lief. 1961. Training for "detached concern" in medical students. In *The psychological basis of medical practice,* ed. Harold Lief, Victor Lief, and Nina Lief. New York: Harper and Row.

Fox, Renee C., and Judith Swazey. 1974. *The courage to fail: A social view of organ transplantation.* Chicago: University of Chicago Press.

———. 1984. Medical morality is not bioethics: Medical ethics in China and the United States. *Perspectives in Medicine and Biology* 27:336–60.

———. 1992. *Spare parts: Organ replacement in American society.* New York: Oxford University Press.

Frader, Joel, and Charles Bosk. 1981. Parent talk at intensive care rounds. *Social Science and Medicine* 15E:267–74.

Gorovitz, Samuel. 1986. Baiting bioethics. *Ethics* 96:356–74.

Grant, Linda, and Daniel DuRose. 1984. Expected rewards of practice and personal life: Priorities of men and women medical students. *Sociological Focus* 17:84–104.

Gray, Bradford H. 1975. *Human subjects in medical experimentation.* New York: John Wiley.

Guillemin, Jean H., and Linda L. Holmstrom. 1986. *Mixed blessings: Intensive care for newborns.* New York: Oxford University Press.

Hafferty, Frederic W. 1991. *Into the valley: Death and the socialization of medical students.* New Haven, Ct.: Yale University Press.

Hilgartner, Steven, and Charles L. Bosk. 1988. The rise and fall of social problems: A public arenas model. *American Journal of Sociology* 94:53–78.

Hoffmaster, Barry. 1992. Can ethnography save the life of medical ethics? *Social Science and Medicine* 35:1421–31.

Knafl, Kathleen and Gary Burkett. 1975. Professional socialization in a surgical specialty: Acquiring medical judgment. *Social Science and Medicine* 9:397–404.

Kuhn, Thomas. 1970. *The structure of scientific revolutions.* 2nd ed. Chicago: University of Chicago Press.

Light, Donald. 1972. Psychiatry and suicide: The management of a mistake. *American Journal of Sociology* 77:821–38.

———. 1975. The sociological calendar: An analytic tool. *American Journal of Sociology* 80:1145–64.

———. 1980. *On becoming psychiatrists.* New York: W. W. Norton.

Lock, Margaret. 2001. *Twice dead.* Berkeley: University of California Press.

Mauss, Marcel. 1967. *The gift.* New York: W. W. Norton.

Merton, Robert K., George Reader, and Patricia Kendall, eds. 1957. *The student-physician.* Cambridge, Ma.: Harvard University Press.

Miller, Steven J. 1970. *Prescription for leadership: Training for the medical elite.* Chicago: Aldine.

Mills, C. Wright. 1959. *The sociological imagination.* New York: Oxford University Press.

Millman, Marcia. 1976. *The unkindest cut: Life in the backrooms of medicine.* New York: Morrow.

Mizrahi, Terry. 1986. *Getting rid of patients: Contradictions in the socialization of physicians.* New Brunswick: Rutgers University Press.

Olesen, Virginia, and Elvi W. Whittaker. 1968. *The silent dialogue: A study on the social psychology of professional socialization.* San Francisco: Jossey-Bass.

Prince, Ellen, Joel Frader, and Charles L. Bosk. 1982. On hedging in physician discourse. In *Linguistics and the professions,* ed. R. J. DiPietro. Norwood, N.J.: Ablex, 83–99.

Putnam, Robert. 2000. *Bowling alone: The collapse and revival of American community.* New York: Simon and Schuster.

Roth, Julius. 1972. Some contingencies of the moral evaluation and control of clientele: The case of the hospital emergency service. *American Journal of Sociology* 77:839–56.

Schneiderman, L. J., T. Gilmer, H. D. Tetzel, D. O. Dugan, J. Blustein, R. Cranford, K. B. Briggs, G. I. Komatsu, P. Goodman-Crews, R. Cohn, and E. W. Young. 2003. Effects of ethics consultation on non-beneficial life-sustaining treatments in the intensive-care setting: A randomized clinical trial. *Journal of the American Medical Association* 290 (6): 1166–72.

Scully, Diana. 1980. *Men who control women's health: The miseducation of obstetrician-gynecologists.* Boston: Houghton Mifflin.

Siegler, Mark. 1979. Clinical ethics and clinical medicine. *Archives of Internal Medicine* 139:914–15.

Simpson, Ida Harper, with Kurt Back. 1979. *From student to nurse: A longitudinal study of socialization.* New York: Cambridge University Press.

Slater, Philip E. 1970. *The pursuit of loneliness: American culture at the breaking point.* Boston: Beacon Press.

Stevens, Tina. 2000. *Bioethics in America: Origins and cultural politics.* Baltimore: Johns Hopkins University Press.

Stinson and Stinson. 1979. The long dying of baby Andrew. *The Atlantic Monthly.*

Sykes, Gresham, and David Matza. 1957. Techniques of neutralization: A theory of delinquency. *American Sociological Review* 22:664–70.

Zerubavel, Eviatar. 1979. *Patterns of time in hospital life.* Chicago: University of Chicago Press.

Zussman, Robert. 1992. *Intensive care: Medical ethics and medical sociology.* Chicago: University of Chicago Press.

Notes

1. One reason for this discomfort that I will not dwell on here is that while I realized that it was fairly easy to state social-science-first principles for an audience largely comprised of non–social scientists without generating much controversy, I was not certain how many of my colleagues would agree with any set of principles that I chose to be dogmatic about. It is hard to imagine those covering laws on which a Marxist, a sociobiologist, and a semiotician agree.

2. The phrase "socially visible activity that we call bioethics" I owe to Charles Rosenberg. It denotes the very large and diverse set of activities that are characterized as bioethics and signals that this collection is quite broad. Typically, characterizations of bioethics emphasize this or that activity but none seem to include the whole set from bedside consulting to armchair theorizing to public policymaking. Nor do these three activities comprise a complete set. They are merely a convenient way of going from the microinteractional to the macrosocial while briefly resting at the solitarily contemplative.

3. I regret that this is so but one of the best ways to get noticed as a social scientist by a bioethicist is to criticize bioethics. Two instructive examples make the point. The first is the response by Gorovitz (1986) to a piece by Fox and Swazey (1984) in the *Hastings Center Report* of which I will have more to say below. The second is the number of critical reviews by bioethicists that Stevens's (2000) history of bioethics provoked.

4. A recent spate of rules regulating the working hours of residents from a staggering variety of national policy-setting bodies has redefined 'total immersion' to eighty hours or double the maximum number that most other labor organizations find acceptable.

5. In commenting on formal rule systems in a different context, Sykes and Matza (1957), in attempting to explain how it was that juveniles broke rules that they were both aware of and believed in, made the claim that a formal property of all systems of rules is incompleteness, incoherence, and internal contradiction. Simply stated knowing a rule is not the same as knowing when to apply it, or knowing which rule to apply when two different rules conflict. What is true for juvenile delinquents is also true for medical workers. Applying rules in situations requires considerable social judgment. Being overly concerned with identifying the correct rule for this situation creates the possibility that we will pay too little attention needed for identifying correctly what this situation is.

6. It is tempting here to claim that if bioethicists had read their Mauss (1967) more carefully they would recognize the concept of the total social

phenomena—one that is at once economic, social, political, and juridical—and that once such a concept is fully appreciated, the bracketing of issues as "ethical" is too crude a form of reductionism to function effectively for thinking about the thorny dilemmas of health care in all their multidimensional complexity.

7. I think this is why virtually all attempts by bioethicists to discuss the absence of universal health insurance in the United States have the quality of non sequiturs.

8. Truth be told, bioethicists do not take so kindly to any of the scolding. As mentioned before, Gorovitz's (1986) response to one of the first scoldings by social scientists (Fox and Swazey 1984) is a nice paradigmatic response of the philosopher's parry to sociologist's thrust. Gorovitz complains that the attack is too general, it paints in broad strokes but provides little in the way of systematic evidence, it pays too little attention to counterexamples, and too little attention to qualifications within a single article. The philosopher's broadside to the sociologists' broadside suggests that, if the sociologists had been more careful scholars, perhaps more like philosophers, they would see that they had no case at all, no complaint to make. Without going into the merits here, perhaps it is enough to say that Gorovitz was insufficiently attuned to Fox and Swazey's use of ideal-type methodology. After all, ideal-types are exaggerations (even distortions, if it is your ox that is being gored) of certain features of a phenomenon that are constructed to allow us to see identifying characteristics more clearly. As Weber never tires of telling us, they never coincide with a particular empirical reality. Somehow this seems like an odd defense for an empirically based discipline to make against charges from a speculative one.

9. If I were either a better field-worker or less guilty about those times that I do step out of role, I would keep a more careful record of them. Instead, I suppress mention of them in my field notes. I do not set out to repress or not record this material. On review, when I have left the field I find it is not there or not there richly enough to become a topic of analysis. This is unfortunate because these role breaches might be an interesting topic for analysis. For example, they might provide a window into the process of empathy in clinical encounters.

10. For me the high-water mark of this distrust and of a rights-based concept of autonomy arrives when commentators on cases involving termination of pregnancy begin to write of the inherent conflict of interest between mother and fetus. In pediatrics, there are also some hurt feelings involved when physicians presume to know better than parents the best interest of severely damaged neonates. These hurt feelings occur on whichever side of the aggressive treatment–treatment withdrawal argument parents of neonates fall (Stinson and Stinson 1979, Bridge and Bridge 1981).

11. To borrow a colorful phrase from the title of an article by Arthur Caplan (1982).

12. At this point I found myself wishing that my department had had a course on field methods and that I had taken it.

Index